# The L.O.V.E. Approach
## to Living with Dementia

### Engaging in life with family and friends!

Vicky Pitner, CTRS, CDP

Copyright © 2024 Vicky Pitner

All rights reserved.

No part of this book may be reproduced, stored in a retrieval system, or transmitted, in any form or by any means, electronic, mechanical, photocopying, recording, or otherwise, without prior written permission from the publisher, except for brief quotations embodied in critical reviews and certain other noncommercial uses permitted by copyright law.

ISBN: 978-1-963949-35-3 (Paperback)

Printed in the United States of America

## Dedication

*To my little sister Tracy, for her love and continued support in helping make my dreams come true.*

## In loving memory

*For my parents, Dot and Red, for their belief in my dreams and the ability to realize them, and to my big sister Pam, for her unconditional love. I miss you all.*

*To Pat Head Summitt for her courage to make a difference in "this disease" and for changing the direction of my life.*

## And a special thank you

*To Marion Walker, who has supported my obsession with this project, brainstormed topics and ideas, listened and provided feedback from the beginning, tolerated my relentless chatter, and always supported the underdogs of the world. But most importantly, for becoming a champion for those living with dementia and advocating for their rights.*

## *About the Book*

Life roles can change so quickly, such as becoming a new parent, resulting in new priorities, responsibilities and commitments. However, when someone you love is diagnosed with a neurocognitive disorder such as Alzheimer's disease or another type of dementia, you may feel you have taken on an unwanted role as a "caregiver." Research has found that many informal "caregivers," such as family members and friends, do not identify with this term and perceive the support and care provided as just part of the responsibility of the relationship. The roles you play in life describe what you do, and your identity is the essence of who you are.

This L.O.V.E. Approach is for family members and friends supporting someone living with dementia at home and offers a deeper understanding of how a dementia diagnosis affects the person and also how it affects you. Developing self-awareness and self-efficacy skills, identifying strengths and believing in yourself helps you gain confidence to make the best decisions and provide optimal care for your loved one.

Recognizing and addressing dementia-related symptoms such as wandering or repetitive storytelling is an attempt to communicate an unmet need such as boredom or loneliness and not a "challenging behavior," fewer conflicts will occur. By practicing how to listen, observe, validate, and engage with your loved one, meaningful relationships can continue and shared joyful experiences are possible.

# Contents

| | | |
|---|---|---|
| | Introduction | 1 |
| Chapter 1 | Pivotal Moments | 3 |
| Chapter 2 | Breaking the Stigma: Shifting the Paradigm of Dementia | 15 |
| Chapter 3 | Engaging in Life | 34 |
| Chapter 4 | The L.O.V.E. Approach: Listen, Observe, Validate, and Engage | 40 |
| Chapter 5 | Meeting Unmet Needs | 56 |
| Chapter 6 | Who am I? Who are you? | 61 |
| Chapter 7 | Self Efficacy | 79 |
| Chapter 8 | A Need for Change | 87 |
| Chapter 9 | Living with Purpose and Meaning | 95 |
| Chapter 10 | Friends, Family and Faith | 108 |
| | Conclusion | 118 |
| | References | 121 |
| | About the Author | 123 |

# *Introduction*

The L.O.V.E Approach for Families and Friends promotes well-being and quality of life by nurturing and creating meaningful relationships with someone living with dementia, especially during the early signs of cognitive decline. By practicing the four simple concepts of Listening, Observing, Validating, and Engaging with your family member or friend, you can experience positive changes in your relationships. Moreover, your loved one will continue to feel purpose and meaning in their life and maintain independence longer.

Using these four concepts will also enhance your ability to listen and understand what the person with dementia is trying to express, observe changes in your and their emotional reactions, validate the person's efforts to express feelings, and become actively engaged in creating a more positive experience/environment for the person with dementia and yourself.

Because of the changes in the brain, a person with dementia cannot physically, cognitively, or emotionally change their communication and comprehensive ability to communicate with us like they used to. However, we can change how we communicate with them by learning new ways to talk, listen, and help them feel valued, loved, and understood.

Learning any new skill takes practice. Enhancing your communication skills to better interact with a person with dementia takes practice and patience, but it is completely worth the effort as interactions will become more pleasant and meaningful, reducing stress for everyone. By gaining a greater awareness of how we talk and listen, relationships are enhanced.

Understanding that people with dementia have difficulty with thinking skills and retaining new information (repeating questions that were just answered) or are unable to retrieve an old memory (such as using a T.V. remote), we can approach the person with more empathy and compassion. Taking the word "remember" out of your vocabulary can reduce the feeling of shame and embarrassment they may go through when they're unable to remember or retrieve information.

If someone has aphasia (an acquired language impairment), the information given may not be received accurately (receptive language), or the person may find difficulty in expressing the information (expressive language) as they are unable to find words, and this creates even more frustration. Imagine the stress you feel when your loved one repeats the same question over and over. Now, just imagine how confused, embarrassed, and ashamed the person feels when they hear, "I already told you," over and over again. In most cases, not only do they forget the answer received earlier, they don't even recall asking the question in the first place. As things stand, it is already very confusing for a person with memory loss to not get answers to simple questions. Now, imagine how this can lead to constant conflicts.

Promoting a quality life for the person living with dementia and their family members and friends is the foundation of the L.O.V.E. Approach. By listening, observing, validating, and engaging in physical activities, intellectual stimulation, socialization, spiritual support, music, and expressive arts, cognitive decline can slow and reduce the frustrations experienced by everyone. Staying engaged with each other is crucial to live a life of quality for the person, their family members, and friends. Ironically, more and more research is showing that cognitive stimulation is not the only treatment approach; continuing to be socially and physically engaging has many benefits. Maintaining these domains in our own lives can help reduce the risk of dementia.

This book is also about helping create a more inclusive society for people living with dementia and their families. The dual stigma of dementia affects the individual and the family and can be the most significant barrier to not seeking a diagnosis and beginning early intervention, which is crucial to the overall outcome of treatment. By utilizing a strength-based and family-centered approach and implementing positivity-focused interventions, engagements in life with the L.O.V.E. Approach will help guide you to become more self-aware, increase your compassion and empathy, giving you the self-efficacy skills to provide love and support for your loved ones with dementia.

# Chapter 1
## *Pivotal Moments*

*"The moment I heard the words, "Your mom has dementia," the air was sucked out of me. I knew my life would change, but at least I knew what we were dealing with.*
*-daughter of a mother diagnosed with dementia*

We all have a story to tell. The collection of pivotal moments that have greatly influenced our lives, such as a new job, moving to another state, a marriage, a death, the birth of a baby, meeting someone new, or learning a loved one has a chronic illness that unexpectedly and abruptly gives pause and reflects on our future. Pivotal moments can help define who we are and can offer insight into how we embrace the changes and challenges of critical moments in our lives.

Pivotal moments can present as "and then" moments and may occur when we least expect them. Those defining moments can be unwanted, and we may feel unprepared. When life changes suddenly, uncertainty, anxiety, stress, and fear can create negative emotions or bring inspiration with the realization of the strengths we never knew we had.

After college, I was working as a therapist in a nursing home in Knoxville, Tennessee, "and then" a friend called me out of the blue to tell me about a job opportunity in Nashville she thought I would love. I left the job in Knoxville, moved to Nashville and began working with adolescents in a rehabilitation facility for addiction. These adolescents were risk takers, so high-risk adventures such as rock climbing and rope course challenges could help satisfy that need for an adrenaline rush. I absolutely loved this work, and after several years, a big unexpected "and then" pivotal moment happened: I sustained a serious work injury that turned my world upside down.

Sometimes, a pivotal moment can change our sense of self, and at the time of my injury, my self-identity did change. The future of my career was in jeopardy, and I would ruminate on my life as an athlete and adventurer and became depressed and began to doubt myself. With the support of family and friends and activating my "superpowers," it became possible for me to develop a new career path that eventually led me to who I am today.

So, what are superpowers? I believe we all have these powers of inner strength that can get us through difficult times. Much like the Superhero who finds the power to defeat the villains, life challenges can present opportunities for growth and inspiration when we find our own unique powers to fight adversity. Did you know the first Superhero, The Phantom, who debuted in a comic strip in 1936, really had no extraordinary superpowers? He was an ordinary man with a wife and two children who relied on his strength and intelligence to fight the forces of evil.

Our "powers" may not be as remarkable and impressive as some Superheroes in movies and comic books, but could it be possible that our powers started before we were born? Spider-Woman's powers of enhanced strength, speed, and an amazing ability to stick to any surface began forming after her mother was struck by radiation while baby Spider-Woman was still in her womb, or Blade's gift of speed as a result of his mother being bitten by a vampire during her pregnancy.

Our personal superpowers are unique and serve us well when we learn how to activate them. So what are superpowers, and why are they important to understand in facing a difficult pivotal moment? Our unique superpowers are the special characteristics that form our personalities and begin to develop when we are young children (or before). These are the characteristics our neighbors, aunts, uncles, friends, parents, teachers, and grandparents used to describe us. These superpowers are not skills we learn throughout the years but our passions, purpose, and inner strengths that have helped us learn skills that help us through life, especially during difficult times. When I began exploring my own superpowers many years ago, I asked my relatives how they saw me as a child: "You were a funny little curious, creative kid." My mother knew my playfulness got me through hard times, and my father recognized my determination to never give up. By tapping in on our own unique talents and gifts, we can awaken the forces within and be able to unleash our own superpowers, restore balance when needed and live a more joyful and satisfying life.

Although we may not think of Dorothy Gale from The Wizard of Oz as having superpowers, she did have powers of inner strength. Unbeknownst to her, by fulfilling a difficult quest to find the Great and Powerful Oz, she realized she had the courage and determination to return home to Kansas, only to discover her happiness was in her own backyard.

Whether things are going well or life becomes challenging, the stronger we are on the inside, the more we can achieve on the outside. Every Superhero will be called on to give their gifts for the greater good. Be ready, give generously, and share your superpowers and gifts with others.

My hope is that by the end of this book, you will learn what makes you tick and realize your inner strengths. The Greek philosopher Socrates said, "To know thyself is the beginning of wisdom." Being willing to know yourself is one of the greatest gifts you can ever have. Reflecting on pivotal moments and patterns in our life, will help you to understand yourself better.

Studies suggest our reactions to negative events in our lives are influenced by the available resources, support from friends and family, the skills we have to regulate our emotions, and the ability to activate our coping skills to manage stress. "In high-stress situations, resources including self-confidence and family support predicted the use of active problem-focused coping." (1)

Another pivotal moment that greatly influenced my life occurred in August of 2011 as I was sitting at my desk in San Francisco. I was working as a private contractor, developing inclusion services for the San Francisco Recreation and Parks Department, "and then" I received a phone call from my sister in Knoxville.

There was no hello. My sister simply began the call with a question. "Did you hear?" I was so surprised to have a call from her in the middle of the day that I didn't even have a response. Her next statement is embedded in my heart forever: "Pat Summit just announced she has Alzheimer's disease." My beloved basketball coach, Pat Head Summit, for the Lady Vols at the University of Tennessee and a pioneer for women's collegiate basketball, just shared a significant "and then" moment with the world. Our hearts were broken.

After I hung up, I searched online to find the announcement. A one-minute and 53-second video shared a life-changing pivotal moment for Pat and her family. Pat was sitting on her sofa at home with her golden retriever by her side, quietly sleeping, with her head on Pat's lap. Coach Summit stoically addressed her Tennessee family and millions of others around the world with the news that she had been diagnosed with early onset Alzheimer's type disease. She was only fifty-nine years old, and I was fifty-five.

Pat Summit was, and still is, an icon in the state of Tennessee. At the time of her diagnosis, she was the winningest NCAA collegiate coach for men and women, transforming women's basketball. On that fall day, her brave announcement became one of my most memorable pivotal moments, both personally and professionally. I wasn't just a fan of Tennessee women's basketball. I was a Lady Vol, and Pat always said, "Once a Lady Vol, always a Lady Vol."

I just couldn't wrap my mind around how Pat, just four years older than me, could have Alzheimer's disease. I first met Pat in 1974 as a walk-on to play basketball at the University of Tennessee in Knoxville. Pat Head was a 22-year graduate student, and I was an 18-year-old freshman. She was a Tennessee basketball star in both high school and college, as well as an Olympian coach and player. She was working on her master's at UT on a graduate assistantship and was hired to be the new coach for the women's basketball team when the former coach retired. I loved basketball and wanted to play.

What I must tell you now is that I was small and scrappy and had only learned to shoot a basketball the summer after graduating from high school by attending two basketball camps. At the time, not all high schools in Tennessee were playing five players. My high school was one that didn't. I was a guard on a six-player team and had no need to develop shooting skills.

Because there were so many young women trying out for the team in 1974, a Junior Varsity team was created. I was thankful because I just wasn't varsity material. We had a great coach who trained us as hard as the varsity team. The JV team lasted a year, and I had a blast. My friend and I had a running joke about our short careers. My friend had three turnovers, and I had three assists, cleaning up the water bottle the three times she knocked it over.

Pat wasn't just a great coach. Her influence on so many lives continues today.

Her decision to share her diagnosis with the world was a remarkable moment for others living with dementia and their families and friends. Her determination to share her news was an intentional effort to increase awareness and help break the stigma of dementia. Shortly after her diagnosis, she and her son Tyler started the Pat Summit Alzheimer's Foundation to advance research and education on Alzheimer's disease. Pat said, "I thought I was going to be remembered for winning basketball games, but I hope I'm remembered for a difference in this disease." When asked how she managed the disease, she calmly stated, "Right foot. Left foot. Breath. Repeat," the same approach she used in coaching to inspire hundreds of young Lady Vols.

At the time of her announcement, I had over 30 years of behavioral healthcare experience under my belt. At different times throughout my career, I created programs for people living with dementia and their families in both clinical and community settings. My work in the 1990s had revolved around serving children with autism and other neurological disorders in community settings, but on that August day, I decided to create my own pivotal moment and focus on gaining a deeper understanding of this disease that eventually took Pat's life in 2016 when she was only sixty-four years old.

What I soon realized that my life experiences, those pivotal moments of job opportunities, my work injury that changed my career path, the people in my life, and my deep compassion to serve others led me to develop the L.O.V.E. Approach for families and friends in supporting someone living with dementia in the home.

Perhaps we share the pivotal moment when our lives became impacted by someone diagnosed with dementia. Was your pivotal moment last year, five years ago, or this week when you began noticing changes in your loved one, and in your heart, you knew something was different? In March of 2023, The World Health Organization estimated that more than 55 million people have dementia worldwide. In the United States, the majority of people, between 70% to 81%, live in their community, and for approximately 75% of these individuals, care is provided by family and friends.

The day my beloved college basketball coach announced to the world that she was diagnosed with early-onset Alzheimer's disease and the day you learned your loved one or friend has dementia impacted both our lives greatly. You decided to care for your loved one at home, and I realized there is insufficient training specific for supporting the families of a loved one.

Learning of the diagnosis can be overwhelming, but also a relief to know what is happening. There are serious consequences of not seeking early intervention services and delaying testing. If you find yourself reluctant to reach out for help, please understand that cognitive decline can be addressed, especially in the early stages. I encourage you to take action today.

Regardless, when you learned your loved one has dementia, the trajectory of your life changed like you never expected. I would imagine you were devastated to learn this unexpected life-changing diagnosis. For any pivotal moment, the choice is always ours in how these life-changing events can change us. Accepting the sadness and grief of a diagnosis of dementia of someone you love is difficult. You may not be able to change the results of the "and then" moment when you realize your life will change, but you have the choice to either embrace it and begin a journey that will support your loved one living with dementia or hide at home and think you can do this on your own. At this moment, you can decide how the next chapter in your story will turn out. With support, self-awareness, and growth, you will hopefully recognize your strengths and gifts. There are big moments and little moments, but a moment of clarity that provides us with a new perspective, a paradigm shift in our thinking, or an opportunity that offers hope can change our lives. Like most people, I've had many. Some moments are more memorable than others. I hope this book will become an "and then" moment for you and perhaps create a shift for you and your family and you can begin living and engaging in life with your family member.

Life can turn around so quickly. When you commit to supporting your family member in the home, you will benefit from specific training designed for your needs, such as believing you can provide quality care and learning how to meet the unmet needs of the behavioral symptoms of dementia. Sometimes, families realize that caring for someone at home is not in the best interest of the person and the family due to the progression of dementia, and that's ok. This book will also support determining the best decision for your family and address the guilt and fear many families experience when transitioning their family members into a memory care community.

As a healthcare professional, I have worked with hundreds of families raising children and young adults with disabilities, including Down syndrome, autism, and other neurocognitive developmental disorders. The saddest statement I hear is when these children tell me they do not have friends. The second saddest statement is when the parent, usually with tears in their eyes, tells me as if it were a confession, "My child doesn't have any friends." Sadly, throughout my years supporting families and their loved ones with dementia, this same statement proved to be true. Because of the lack of initiation with a person with dementia, a common dementia-related symptom, it is up to you to help create a circle of support and include old and new friends to avoid the loneliness and isolation that a diagnosis can bring.

I hope you enjoy this book. It offers opportunities to develop self-awareness, expand your knowledge, and help you achieve personal growth while supporting a loved one living with dementia. It also offers you a deeper understanding of how a dementia diagnosis is affecting you and your family. The book reflects on experiences from my work as a therapist, encouraging people to gain confidence and self-determination to make positive decisions and how this relates to their situations. I am straightforward and believe we need to stop walking on an eggshell sidewalk and bring awareness to sensitive issues that are not being addressed.

I believe this book will make a difference in your life and in the person you love because I have seen it work with hundreds of families throughout the years. If you are supporting a family member or friend with memory loss in the home, the practical and evidence-based strategies throughout the chapters will help you experience connectedness, maintain meaningful relationships and create moments of joy with the person you care about.

It is not easy supporting someone living with memory loss and the progression of changes in the brain but learning to identify the person's unmet needs and how to address them to minimize dementia-related symptoms can assist you in establishing goals and priorities to feel successful. Much like you, I continue to have "and then" moments that influence my life. Some have not been pleasant, and it took time for me to understand why that event or person came into my life, but I have always had a new "and then" experience or new people in my life, and a wonderful "and then" moment presents itself.

I believe we create our own pivotal moment to promote a positive change when a negative change happens. Creating our destinies and not allowing circumstances or events to define our lives when a critical life-changing event occurs. When we come to a "fork in the road," and we realize our lives will never be the same, should we live with magical thinking (I just wish he could remember again) or dig deep in our souls and activate our superpowers and create a positive pivotal moment?

You hold the power to decide how the next chapters in your life story are written. I always encourage families who have a loved one with dementia not to let a crisis or an event make the decisions for them. Too often, families will muddle through this journey with little planning or preparation for the future for their families. With appropriate training for family members, learning new communication strategies and living an engaged life after a dementia diagnosis is possible. Staying connected in social and physical activities, sharing meaningful activities, and offering opportunities for self-expression, is a well-rounded approach to reaping the benefits of the positive aspects of supporting someone living with dementia. Learning how and why to keep your family member or friend with dementia active and engaged in the community encourages purpose and well-being for the person and for the family and friends. The worse possible scenario is for you and your family member to isolate and be disconnected from friends and neighbors. Social isolation is associated with faster cognitive decline, depression, and stress for the entire family. On the other hand, staying active is associated with a reduced risk of cognitive decline and depression, not just for the person but for those providing constant care.

How do you understand your life-changing events? I hope this book can be a part of your next "and then" moment and support you as you support your friend or family member living at home. I am confident that this unique, innovative, and family and friends strengths-based approach will empower you to make the changes necessary to promote a life of quality and well-being for you and your family.

*"When a defining moment comes along, you define the moment, or the moment defines you."*
-Kevin Costner.

## Activity 1

## Identifying Your Superpowers

Our "Superpowers" are the strengths and unique gifts we use to problem-solve and manage our emotions.

Think back to the character traits your family and friends used to describe when you were young. Were you perseverant, courageous, fearless, kind, adventurous, spunky, or confident?

Write your superpowers and unique gifts in the space below.

# Activity 2

## Connecting the Dots

1. Close your eyes and imagine a meaningful moment in your life that brought you great joy.

2. Now make a list of books you have read that had an influence in your life and write them in the space below.

3. Think about people who have greatly influenced your life. Who are they?

# Activity 3

## Pivotal moments and how I addressed them

Reflect on three difficult, life-changing events and identify your character strengths to overcome the challenge.

Year _____ Event _____

Character strengths you use _____

Something I wish I had done differently _____


Year _____ Event _____

Character strengths _____

Something I wish I had done differently _____


Year _____ Event _____

Character strengths _____

Something I wish I had done differently _____

# Activity 4

## Pre-evaluation of knowledge, awareness, attitudes, and values. Please circle the response that best describes you.

1. Understanding dementia is      poor    fair    good    great

2. Ability to care for my loved one      poor    fair    good    great

3. Skills needed to provide care      poor    fair    good    great

4. Confidence to provide care      poor    fair    good    great

5. The belief I need to learn new skills      poor    fair    good    great

6. Importance of my needs      poor    fair    good    great

7. My motivation to change      poor    fair    good    great

8. I value myself, and my needs      poor    fair    good    great

9. Knowledge of dementia symptoms      poor    fair    good    great

10. Believe that recreation is important      poor    fair    good    great

11. Confidence this book will help me      poor    fair    good    great

12. My social support is      poor    fair    good    great

Notes

# Notes

## Chapter 2
## Breaking the Stigma: Shifting the Paradigm of Dementia

*"When my husband's behaviors began to change, I thought he was having an affair."*
-*Spouse of a man diagnosed with frontotemporal dementia*

Deciding to care for a loved one living with dementia in the home comes with great responsibility. There is an expectation of trust from the person with dementia that they will receive appropriate medical care and be involved in the decision-making as long as the person is able. Personal decisions such as food preferences, clothes to wear, and places to go will help maintain dignity and autonomy. Providing opportunities to have positive human contact and socialize, stay physically active, participate in hobbies or other meaningful activities, and offer options for self-expression, and spiritual expression is a basic human right.

In order to provide the best care for your family member, you must understand and address the specific needs a dementia diagnosis brings. With proper training and support, families can create a safe and loving environment, which is crucial to promote quality of life and overall well-being for both the person living with memory loss and the family. This approach will keep the person independent longer, and as unmet needs are identified and addressed, you and your loved one can enjoy less stressful interactions. The L.O.V.E Approach encompasses a holistic framework to focus on the lived experiences of the person and address the whole person.

Studies are readily available to identify the different aspects of providing support for a loved one with memory loss, including dementia-related behavioral symptoms and communication challenges due to confusion and anxiety. These behaviors are usually the person trying to express an unmet need. If the person thinks someone is stealing money, it may be they forgot where their wallet or purse is. Helping search for these items can relieve that fear, especially when they discover a small sum of money in the lost item affords the person dignity. These symptoms are not present when supporting someone with other chronic illnesses. Research does indicate that supporting someone with dementia does take specialized training for the family in order to provide the support their family member requires.

A recent study published in the National Library of Medicine shows that with self-efficacy training, an in-depth understanding of the dementia-related behavioral symptoms, a shift in beliefs about people living with dementia, advocation for the person, self-care, and utilizing effective psychosocial interventions, family members and friends can have a more positive experience while supporting the family member at home. Other factors that can determine the positive outcome of support at home are the satisfaction, rewards, and personal growth of the family members.

Factors that can result in either a negative or positive experience of supporting a family member at home are the relationships of the family members prior to the diagnosis, the understanding and knowledge the family has about dementia, the willingness to learn positive interactions, resilience of the family, motive for home support, and the current family circumstances.

Programs that promote the positive aspects of supporting someone with dementia that offer dyadic interactions between the person with dementia and a family member to encourage the connectedness the two can share are growing. Also, by taking a whole-body approach, positive aspects of support can be enhanced. The L.O.V.E. Approach trainings offer all of these interventions. With training specifically for family members and friends supporting someone at home, including learning new communication strategies and observation skills to identify and meet unmet needs, there are more positive outcomes, and the person can remain independent longer.

Staying engaged in social and physical activities, cognitive stimulation, providing opportunities for self-expression, and meeting the spiritual needs of the person living with dementia are possible using a holistic and eco-psychosocial approach. Learning how to support your family member to live with dementia positively includes keeping you, your family, and your family member or friend with dementia active and engaged in the community. The worse possible scenario is for you and your family member to isolate and become disconnected from friends and neighbors. Social isolation is associated with faster cognitive decline, depression and increased stress for the entire family. On the other hand, staying active and socially engaged is associated with a reduced risk of cognitive decline and depression.

There are so many misconceptions about Alzheimer's disease, dementia, and aging. The stereotypical depiction and "stigma" that portrays people with dementia as "crazy" or not even a whole person prevents individuals and families from seeking help. According to the Britannica Dictionary, a stigma is a set of negative and unfair beliefs that a society or group of people have about something. Stigmatizing people with dementia results in individuals being judged and discriminated against. Thus, the projected outcome of a dementia diagnosis is portrayed as negative, often by both the healthcare providers and the family.

Despite the advances in research and efforts to raise more education and awareness, the stigma of dementia hasn't seemed to have changed much over the 40 years I have been a clinician. People still see those with dementia and Alzheimer's disease as "suffering." Family members and friends do suffer as they watch the changes in someone they love, but with a proper diagnosis and a more holistic approach to addressing the unmet needs, a person with dementia can live a life of quality. Engaging in life with the L.O.V.E. Approach encourages people to shift their previous beliefs and begin seeing someone with memory loss as "living with dementia" and recognizing their strengths and gifts to ensure they maintain their personhood and dignity.

As we age, we may fear losing our independence with changes in functioning abilities. The anxiety and stress of aging are referred to as "ageism," or a stereotypic belief in how we think about older people needs to be examined. The World Health Organization reports, "Ageism can change how we view ourselves, can erode solidarity between generations, can devalue or limit our ability to benefit from what younger and older populations can contribute." Older workers may be perceived as unsuitable for tasks that are commonly associated with younger workers and may cause a reduction in self-esteem and motivation. Older adults in general experience a stigma of aging and may experience discrimination, especially in the workforce." We all may experience some decline in our physical and cognitive health as we get older, but the good news is that studies show that happiness actually increases with age! (2)

Our efforts to maintain a positive attitude and feel good about ourselves by staying fit and healthy as we grow older can be sabotaged by common myths about aging and prevent us from living life to the fullest. Many people make assumptions about aging and what it is like to "grow old"; however, aging does not have to cause worry or dread. There has been much research on how to manage good health, and studies continue to show that having friends and avoiding social isolation is important to minimize the risk of depression, dementia and so many other health issues.

Maintaining our health by staying active, eating well, engaging in hobbies, socializing, cognitive stimulation by learning, and getting the proper amount of sleep are the recommendations for aging well and reducing the risks of developing dementia. Ironically, these same suggestions are effective in living well with dementia.

One of the most common misunderstandings about aging is that developing dementia is inevitable. Let me be clear. Dementia and Alzheimer's disease are not part of normal aging, although risks can increase as you get older. The stigma of dementia is perpetuated by so many misconceptions, such as the mispronunciation of "Alzheimer's" referring to the disease "All Timers" or "Old Timers."

The World Health Organization reports, "Dementia is not a disease but rather a broad umbrella term used to describe a group of symptoms that affects daily activities of living." Dementia is a progressive neurological disorder, and some people may present with a combination or mixed dementia. Regardless of which dementia the person has, each person will experience dementia in their own unique way.

Symptoms can affect thinking skills, memory, language, changes in mood, and cognitive decline. Alzheimer's disease is the leading cause of dementia. Other causes of dementia include early-onset Alzheimer's disease, vascular dementia, dementia with Lewy bodies, and frontotemporal dementia. Huntington's disease, Creutzfeldt-Jakob disease, Parkinson's disease, alcohol-related dementia, HIV-associated neurocognitive disorder, and multiple sclerosis are other causes of dementia.

Missing appointments or misplacing items can be signs of forgetfulness. However, forgetfulness and memory loss are not the same. The stigma of Alzheimer's disease and dementia, much like with mental illness and addiction, has a double stigma. Not only do the family and friends experience the public stigma with the negative reactions and prejudices, but harmful emotional consequences of self-stigma can also cause a lack of confidence in the individual, creating self-doubt and poor self-image, and the person may respond by self-isolating.

Forgetfulness is a common characteristic of aging, but are forgetful people prone to dementia? Not necessarily because we can all be forgetful. How often do you walk into a room and forget why you are there? Giving yourself a few seconds to concentrate or even walking out of the room and returning can help "jog" your memory. As we age, the speed we process information can slow, but if we misplace our glasses or forget someone's name, eventually, the person's name will "pop" in our head, and we will soon recall where we left the glasses. This is normal aging.

However, persons who are experiencing memory loss may misplace their glasses, and if they do eventually find them, they may not be able to recall their function. An evaluation to determine if something more serious is developing is critical. The actions (or lack of actions) that friends and family members take when they recognize significant changes in a person's thinking and memory reflect directly on the outcome of the person's future. Sadly, the Word Alzheimer's Report in 2021 estimates that "75% of all dementia cases go undiagnosed across the globe, and up to 90 percent in low-middle-income -countries."

If you do have concerns about any cognitive changes in a loved one or friend, you have a couple of options. You can either embrace the person and help them seek professional guidance so they can understand what is happening, and you can learn how to support the person, or you can ignore your concerns and protect yourself from the truth. Denial is useful to delay something that is painful, especially if your life will be affected by the outcome. However, when denial interferes with the well-being of our loved ones, the outcome can be devastating.

Preparing to address your concerns takes some planning. Much like interventions that are created to motivate someone to seek help if they are abusing alcohol or other drugs, seeking out a dementia expert to assist with the strategies to talk to your loved one or friend is very helpful. The earlier the concerns are addressed, the person's ability to maintain independence and live a life with meaning increases. Would it make sense to deny concerns if you noticed a physical change in your friend or family member, such as a new limp or change in a mole?

Facing the stigma of dementia is a primary concern for people living with Alzheimer's disease and their families. Our beliefs determine our actions. Keeping you and your family member active in the community is very important to reduce the loneliness that dementia can bring and help break the stigma of negative attitudes and discrimination. Staying connected with others improves the overall quality of life not only for the person with dementia but also for the family and friends.

Fear and misinformation are two reasons people delay a visit to a healthcare professional. Despite the heroic efforts to raise awareness and help break the stigma of dementia by many public figures like Pat Summit, Tony Bennett, Glen Campbell, Robin Williams and most recently, Bruce Willis, dementia is the second most feared illness, just behind cancer. (3)

After Glen Campbell's death in 2017, I heard Kim Campbell, his wife, speak about their journey living with Alzheimer's disease. One story she shared was about when he attended a day program for people with memory loss. She shared hesitations for him to attend but thought he would enjoy the socialization. The first morning, she gave him several guitar picks to keep in his pocket, thinking this might bring him comfort.

When Kim picked him up, she was a bit leery of asking about his day, but staff happily reported that Glen was going around the center shaking hands, introducing himself, and handing out the picks, just as he had done at his Meet and Greets for years! This was a wonderful example of continuing to help her husband maintain dignity and purpose in his life. Much like Glen's guitar picks, it is soothing for all people to have items with them that provide some level of comfort, especially for those with dementia.

It is important to respect the needs of those with dementia. I was consulting with an adult day program, and one of the women brought her purse with her wallet, family photos, costume jewelry, tissues, a small stuffed animal, and other items she could rummage through when anxious. However, the director insisted the purse be placed in the woman's assigned "box" during the day to keep it "safe." Of course, this was explained to the woman every morning upon arrival, but when she felt anxious or confused, she would retrieve her purse, and staff would immediately return it to the "safety" of her box.

This constant attempt to control this woman's need to have her handbag and the continued emphasis on the "safety" of her purse created more fear and compulsions for her need to check on the purse many times throughout the day. Purses are very important to women. A purse is not only an essential accessory item that most women carry through their adulthood, but it also holds emotional meanings and a sense of personhood. I observed her leave a group to check on her purse and attempt to bring it with her, only to have staff return it to the box for "safety." I suggested to the director to allow the woman to keep her purse with her but was told, "It is against the rules." The director pointed out that she might lose it or not pay attention during activities. I was pretty insistent (reminding her she had hired me to consult), so the director finally agreed to try the strategy for a few days. Did the woman lose or misplace the purse, you ask? Of course not. The woman never let it get out of her sight and sat proudly in groups with her purse safely on her lap and happily participated in the activities with no anxiety, agitation or obsessive thoughts.

After college, at the age of 22, I was a young punk full of energy and ready to change the world. My first job was in a nursing home, where I was introduced to the realities of dementia. But unfortunately, I was not prepared for the exclusion and isolation of persons living with dementia. But at that time, over forty years ago, dementia was seen as a hopeless and terrifying illness and offered little understanding or support for families. The treatment approach at that time was to admit the person with memory loss and other dementia-related symptoms to a nursing home for "pharmacology interventions" and "reality therapy." Many of the patients were physically restrained or heavily medications to keep them "safe" and not wander about in an attempt to "manage" dementia-related behaviors.

Of course, that only caused frustrations, shame, and anger from the person, and they were confused and scared and were expected to remember when they couldn't. The staff didn't understand a person who could not store memories any longer cannot retrieve a memory that didn't store. Even as a young adult, I knew this was not fair or effective, but I was lost on how to comfort these individuals.

Often, they were overmedicated and were too tired or sleepy to enjoy any of the activities that were offered that could possibly bring them joy. Unfortunately, over-medicating persons with dementia-related behaviors, rather than addressing the unmet needs of the person, is still common today, even for those living at home.

Reality therapy is an attempt to make the patients remember current information, such as the day, month, and year. Large calendars, clocks and the name of the facility were strategically placed on the wall in each room directly in front of the person's bed in hopes this would help them to "remember." And if that wasn't confusing enough for a confused person sitting in bed much of the day to all day, staff called attention to the wall each time they entered the room and "reminded" them where they were and the day of the month. Constantly correcting a person who cannot remember causes arguments as the person may believe that they were at their son's house and it was Christmas Day, although it might be the middle of July.

If you visited a grandparent or parent in a nursing facility 40 years ago, you might have the same images I recall. People continue to talk about the dismal settings and ineffective care in the past, which perpetuate the stigma and fears of transitioning a family member into any memory care community. It is much different today, and by developing advocacy skills, selecting the right community for your family, and continuing to engage with your family member, a memory community can be a viable option when caring for your loved one at home is no longer serving their needs.

By the 1980s, Naomi Feil, a German gerontologist, introduced "Validation therapy," a holistic approach for more effective communication that helped change the treatment for persons with dementia. She discovered as a young child during her time spent in a "home for the aged" where her father was the administrator, and her mother was a social worker, that by validating the reality of a severely disoriented person rather than imposing a different reality, the person was much happier and engagement was possible. Going with the flow and engaging in their world is effective and, with practice, becomes quite easy and fun as you connect with the person.

After the 1990s, modern senior assisted living communities were introduced, and quality of care became the top priority. Memory care communities soon followed to provide a safe environment to meet the specific needs of those with dementia. As with any retirement community or assisted living community, you may want to consider exploring for future planning and for emergencies.

Many memory care communities offer "respite weekends," and this is a great option for the family to rejuvenate while your family member is safe. Financial resources are always a concern, but if you are able to use a home health agency or private carer to provide respite one or two days a week, it will give you an opportunity to practice self-care, and your family member will begin to acclimate to having support other than from you.

I encourage all families not to allow an unplanned circumstance or event to make decisions for them. Family members, especially spouses caring for someone with dementia living at home, are at risk for health issues due to the stress of necessary constant support. From my experience, families rarely have an emergency "action plan" in place if an unexpected hospitalization or crisis occurs and the primary support person is suddenly unavailable. This happened recently to a family I was coaching when an unexpected event happened. The mother was supporting her husband at home, and when she suddenly became ill, her sons had no choice but to hospitalize their dad for a week while they sought a solution for his care.

One day, while working at the nursing home, I passed a man's room, and he called out to me. I could see he was seated in a large chair with a restraint around his waist, preventing him from getting up. He whispered as if he knew he shouldn't be asking for any help. "And then," he looked at me straight into my eyes and clearly stated, "Sister, if you can find a pair of scissors, I believe we can get out of here."

And I did. Sadly I had to leave him, but shortly after that defining moment of clarity and realizing that morally and ethically, my values were conflicted, I left the job only after a few months. "And then," I received the call that shifted my career to working with adolescents and adults recovering from substance abuse. Please note: My experience in that nursing home was specific to me and that particular nursing home and perhaps only an example of the lack of understanding of dementia at that time.

My ineffective skills and the overwhelming fears I had in that first job pails in comparison to the techniques and engagement strategies I practiced 44 years later. To my delight, if a person experiencing confusion tells me it is Christmas Day in the middle of July, I get as excited as they do! I whip out my phone with my holiday playlist, and we belt out a duet of Christmas carols with great enthusiasm and share a joyful moment. What harm is in that? By validating the person's reality, the person feels valued but, most importantly, heard and understood. This approach shows compassion and respect, and by stepping into the person's world, a positive connection evolves, and a conflict can be avoided by trying to convince the person Christmas is five months away.

Many family and friends struggle with this approach as they feel they are lying to their family members, wanting to correct the person. But what is really important for someone living in a different reality? Facts are no longer relevant to them. Focusing on their feelings, well-being and connectedness becomes more important. It is just a kinder approach and a more effective means of positive communication. There are times when you need to be truthful depending on their capacity to process the information, but if you need to be "the constant corrector" (here comes a direct shot from my hip), then you are the problem. Changing your behavior is difficult, but creating an environment that promotes not just physical safety but emotional safety can help reduce your loved one's stress and anxiety.

In early 2000, I became a Parent Educator, teaching the importance of setting limits and boundaries with children in order to raise a self-reliant child. A young mom called to schedule a parenting class for redirecting a child's behavior. She told me she had a five-year-old and a two-year-old and wanted to know if her two-year-old was too young to attend. I explained that the children did not attend and the only way we can change a child's behavior is to change our own.

She was a bit shocked and disappointed, to say the least when she realized it was her behavior that needed redirecting, such as the way she spoke, reasoned or interacted with her child. Please note: This story does not reflect in any way that adults with dementia should ever be treated as a child. It only demonstrates that our behaviors must change, as our family member with dementia cannot change their behaviors. Always use respect, adult activities, and language (avoid "baby ease" or "baby talk") when speaking to any adult.

## Breaking the Stigma of Dementia

Imagine waking up in the morning confused and not recognizing where you are. Imagine walking out of the bedroom, and your daughter appears and immediately questions why you are not dressed. Your daughter, who you might not recognize at first, immediately begins to "remind" you of the doctor's appointment that you have been told about several times, even as recently as last night. Imagine you are unable to retain new information and did not know of the appointment, so imagine now how you might respond. Now, imagine you have dementia.

You likely would deny knowing about the appointment or even argue that you do not need to see a doctor as you feel fine. Continue to imagine how this interaction can become intense, and both you and your daughter begin to argue. Imagine the shame you feel because you didn't remember the appointment and the fear you feel about seeing a doctor you don't need. Imagine the emotional pain you feel because you want your daughter to feel the same emotions as you.

This is a simple example of what a person living with dementia may feel when they are experiencing confusion. Likely, the above scenario led to a conflict that lasted all morning, and the appointment possibly had to be canceled. Being able to show deep empathy and compassion for a person with dementia results in outcomes that are much more productive and pleasant. By being able to connect to the person and feel their emotion, you can better understand and interact more calmly and effectively.

It is not always easy. Practicing to understand the person's emotions will result in better relationships, less arguing, and a shared and meaningful connection. So, let's try this same scene again but using a different approach. Imagine your father wandering out of the bedroom, waking up confused and not recognizing where he is. Imagine you greeting him with a warm smile and a cheerful "Good morning, Dad." Imagine inviting him to join you in the kitchen for coffee, and when you notice his hesitation, you slowly walk up to him and reach out your arm. Imagine his smile as he gently places his hand under your elbow. As you walk toward the kitchen, imagine the relief on his face as you assure him who you are and ask, "Have I told you I love you today?"

Now imagine watching your dad become calm and comfortable as he sits at the kitchen table and eases into his morning routine. Imagine touching his hand and smiling as he sips on his coffee rather than "reminding him of the doctor's appointment." Imagine telling him of the appointment but apologizing to him for not letting him know sooner. You assure him there is plenty of time to get dressed, make it to the appointment on time, and even eat breakfast at his favorite restaurant. Then imagine you asking how he feels about that. Imagine you listening as he speaks. Lastly, imagine how validated, understood, and loved your father felt because you made an effort to be patient and show empathy to understand the fear and confusion he was feeling.

Perspective taking, or "putting yourself in the shoes of the person with a stigma" (first example above) and "imagined contact," imagining interaction with the person with the stigma (second example), are prejudice-reducing strategies and shows promise to help decrease the stigma of mental illness, homelessness, and obesity. Two studies at the University of British Columbia suggest "imagined contact is a more promising technique for reducing stigma against depression than perspective-taking."

The study suggests that different prejudice reduction strategies should be used for different stigmatized groups. (4) I was unable to find a study specific to dementia, but why wouldn't it work to help change the stigma of dementia?

People living with dementia still have emotions, feelings, observations, insights, and opinions, but when we discount the person and take away their dignity because we have a certain agenda (get to the doctor's appointment) rather than go with their agenda (wake up slow and needing the reassurance of trust and safety), the days will become less stressful, and relationships can be more meaningful.

Efforts by the medical profession to address the stigma of dementia were published by the American Psychiatric Association in the fifth edition of the Diagnostic and Statistical Manual (DSM 5) in 2013. Replacing the word "dementia" with "Neurocognitive disorders" and defining it as a general term that describes decreased mental function due to a medical disease other than a psychiatric illness. It is often used synonymously but incorrectly with dementia. Dementia is now referred to as one of the characteristics below.

## Mild Neurocognitive Disorders

Mild Cognitive Impairment (MCI) is considered a Mild Neurocognitive Disorder. Some adults do have more memory or thinking problems than others, such as forgetting appointments, misplacing items, forgetting to take important medications, or having trouble finding familiar words or names of familiar people. Mild cognitive impairment (MCI) was initially conceptualized as a transitional zone between normal aging and dementia; however, Mild Cognitive Impairment (MCI) is not dementia. Rather, it is a condition that affects thinking problems and some memory issues, but the person can carry out daily routines and care for themselves. Approximately 10% to 20% of people over age 65 currently have MCI. There are no personality changes in the person, and compensatory skills can be learned, such as keeping notes, following a routine, carrying a pocket calendar, and setting timers for appointments or as medication reminders. People who are diagnosed with MCI have more difficulty with some daily tasks than other people their age, and in many cases, these symptoms can remain stable for several years.

However, according to the 2022 edition of *the Alzheimer's Association Disease and Facts and Figures* special report, *More Than Normal Aging: Understanding Mild Cognitive Impairments,* approximately 12% to 18% of people 60 years or older living with MCI will develop Alzheimer's disease.

There is a portion of employed adults that may experience difficulties with work-related activities or have reduced workability due to early on-set dementia or MCI; worldwide, it is, in fact, estimated that 10% of the 35.6 million people living with some form of cognitive decline are under the age of 65. (5)

A large percentage of people living with MCI that begins to manifest into Alzheimer's disease are undiagnosed, and this can result in serious safety concerns. They continue to drive, make mistakes with their medications, and may not be eating or keeping up with activities of daily living such as hygiene and keeping a safe home. They are at high risk of getting lost or becoming vulnerable to fraud and financial scams. Many are living alone, but those living with a family member may make excuses for these behaviors, contributing to "old age."

A study by Patricia Boyle at the Rush Alzheimer's Disease Research Center in Chicago shows that seniors who are "less likely to detect a scam" may be an early sign of dementia. For example, difficulty managing money and making sound financial decisions could be an early sign of cognitive decline.

A traumatic brain injury (TBI) can also be considered a neurological disorder, depending on the severity of the TBI. Compensatory skills can be taught to help keep up with appointments and important information, much like mild cognitive impairment (MCI). A TBI can be on a continuum and move into a Major Neurocognitive Disorder cognitive.

Several years ago, a friend was a counselor in an outpatient TBI Rehab program and introduced me to a man with a traumatic brain injury. Wayne (not his real name) was a recreation therapist prior to his injury and was graduating from the TBI program and would be looking for employment. She knew I was hiring camp counselors for a therapeutic day camp and referred him to me. He set up an interview and was offered a job and was thrilled for an opportunity to work in the field he loved again.

His TBI affected his short-term memory, and because he had a disability, he requested "reasonable accommodations" according to the guidelines of the ADA. These simple accommodations were to ensure successful employment. He carried a written camp schedule at all times and was encouraged with reminders of assigned tasks with clear expectations. He was given written notes from meetings, and we kept the line of communication open. Staff were also provided additional training and thus easily supported Wayne as a team member.

I tell this story because, despite a cognitive disability, Wayne was able to work with support and reasonable accommodations. Most often, people who begin showing signs of difficulty performing familiar tasks due to a cognitive issue, instead of attempting to work with the employee, the person is "encouraged" to take "early retirement" or worse, forced out with a termination. You may know someone that this happened to.

According to the Equal Employment Opportunity Commission (EEOC), " Ideally, employees will request a reasonable accommodation before the performance or conduct problems arise, or at least before they become too serious." If you or a loved one finds yourself in a situation where accommodations would be helpful to continue working, I recommend you contact the Equal Employment Opportunity Commission (EEOC). A diagnosis is necessary to pursue this option, but I think many individuals I have worked with could have continued to work longer with a reasonable accommodation.

Wayne was a valued employee and co-worker who worked at the camp for several summers and was a great employee. He was a gentle giant, and the children adored him, and he developed positive peer relationships. His dedication to his job and his determination to succeed was relentless. One morning, Wayne called to tell me he would be late because he had car trouble. Unbeknownst to me, a U-Haul rental store was within walking distance of his apartment. Fifteen minutes after I got the call that he would be late, he came rolling up a 16' U-Haul and walked into camp as if nothing was unusual. We can never underestimate the abilities of people.

## Major Neurocognitive Disorders (MND)

Major Neurocognitive Disorders (MND) are described as a substantial decline in function (loss of independence) as a result of profound cognitive impairment. This includes Alzheimer's disease, early-onset Alzheimer's disease, Lewy Body disease, vascular dementia, and frontotemporal dementia. Other causes of dementia can be severe Traumatic Brain Injury (TBI) and alcohol-related dementia. If the functioning level of MCI changes and causes a progressive decline in memory, reasoning, social skills, and emotional reactions, and these deficits are severe enough to impact daily functioning, it is considered to be a Major Neurocognitive Disorder or MND.

Paying attention to lapses in memory of your loved one will be helpful when discussing with the doctor at the appointment. Be mindful that your family member still understands when he/she is being talked about and feels shame and embarrassment. Be thoughtful about how you speak with the physician when your loved one is present. The person will likely deny there are any issues with thinking, problem-solving or memory, so observations you can share with the doctor will assist in receiving early support and the need to do formal testing.

## Dementia

The Center for Disease Control and Prevention (CDC) defines dementia as a "general term for the impaired ability to remember, think, or make decisions that interfere with doing everyday activities." Alzheimer's disease is the most common type of dementia.

As mentioned earlier, a common myth is that memory loss is a part of normal aging. This is not true, and people experiencing early signs of dementia may miss out on early interventions that can begin with a proper diagnosis. Often, the family member is aware of the memory issues and will compensate with humor or "catchphrases," and the diagnosis is missed or delayed.

Below are some early signs that could warrant a dementia screening:

- Unable to store memories. Your family member cannot recall what he/she ate for breakfast, for example. Difficulty with short-term memory

- Difficult to focus, reason, and pay attention, even for short periods of time.

- Receptive (information they hear) and expressive (words they speak) challenges when communicating.

- Visual perception can be affected.

- Getting lost in a familiar neighborhood, either walking or driving.

- Difficulty finding words or using unusual words to refer to something.

- Being repetitive with stories or asking the same question over and over.

- Beginning to struggle using the microwave, television remote or cell phone.

We must improve our efforts to raise awareness and provide education to understand dementia so individuals and families can receive the proper diagnosis and treatment early on. Recently, I was consulting for a company with eight group homes that served people with developmental and intellectual disabilities, including adults with Down syndrome. I was called to address a situation that arose and was asked to "develop a behavior plan" for a 52-year-old man with Down syndrome who was repeatedly losing his wallet. Staff reported they found it in the refrigerator, another time in the staff office, and various other places and were frustrated as the man continually inquired about his lost wallet.

He was also going into other residents' rooms and searching through their dresser drawers and closets, and the staff was unable to stop this behavior. I met with this gentleman and, after a brief conversation, recommended a dementia and geriatric depression screening. Depression can mimic dementia-related behaviors, and it was important to rule out depression. The outcome of the testing did indicate early—onset Alzheimer's disease. The staff received training on effective and appropriate strategies to ensure the gentleman could remain in the group home with his friends. This is an example of the need for awareness of dementia and the higher risk for adults with Down syndrome. The staff was treating this as a "behavior management" issue and not seeing his behavior had a purpose and providing the man the proper care for his dementia.

The Alzheimer's Association reports adults with Down syndrome are at a higher risk for developing Alzheimer's disease as early as their 40s or 50s. According to the National Down Syndrome Society, about 30% of people with Down syndrome who are in their 50s have Alzheimer's disease. **More awareness and better training of our healthcare professionals could certainly increase the chances of recognizing dementia earlier and providing timely treatment.**

Several years ago, I noticed symptoms of late afternoon confusion and disorientation in my 17-year-old Maltese dog. Her behaviors were much like the "Sundowners Syndrome" phenomenon in a person with dementia, such as late afternoon confusion, restlessness, agitation, and wandering.

Thankfully, Savanah's veterinarian was familiar with these symptoms and diagnosed her with Caine Cognitive Decline (CCD) or "Doggie Dementia." I was grateful I had the awareness to recognize signs of cognitive decline with my dog, although I had never heard of CCD. With a proper diagnosis, she was prescribed CBD drops for her water bowl to reduce her anxiety, and I began a robust exercise routine and incorporated stimulating activities that allowed her to remain curious and playful until her death six months later.

## Bio-Medical Approach to Treatment

When someone recognizes changes in thinking and is experiencing memory lapses, the person and their family are often relieved there is a medical cause. If the diagnosis indicates a neurocognitive disorder, the "bio-medical model" focuses on what is "wrong" with the person; the treatment begins by treating the brain with medication, not considering the lived experiences of the person or the family's needs, other than perhaps suggesting the family to attend a support group.

Sadly, many healthcare professionals have low expectations of the overall outcomes of a dementia diagnosis, and rarely do they encourage individuals, families, or friends to explore alternative treatment options. Also, scheduling an appointment for initial testing could be three to six months out. Usually, a follow-up appointment is scheduled six months to a year later to retest and report the changes in the brain and make medication changes. To me, that does not give much hope to these families. Medication is prescribed to treat symptoms of dementia, such as depression, anxiety, sleep difficulties, or confusion. Unfortunately, the drugs that are prescribed to address the symptom can have unpleasant side effects such as nausea, vomiting, a rash, muscle pain or loss of appetite. So is it fair to have a loved one experience these possible side effects so we can "manage their behaviors," or should we explore other ways to address concerning behaviors?

I am not anti-drug therapy, but I believe that bridging models of care and utilizing holistic approaches to address symptoms of dementia-related behaviors can result in a more comprehensive approach to supporting your friend or loved one with dementia.

## An Eco-psychosocial Approach to Treatment

Eco-psychosocial interventions focus on learning communication techniques, teaching strategies for connectedness and engagement, and using a whole-body approach by addressing the environment and staying active in the community and meeting the physical, cognitive, social, expressive and spiritual needs of the person and the family. Interventions can include museums, music, exercise, visual arts, reminiscent therapy, validation therapy and tapping into hobbies and meaningful activities.

By embracing new methods to treat persons living with Alzheimer's disease or another type of dementia, the eco-psychosocial approach focuses on the social environment and the psychosocial needs of the person and their relationships. The interactions and how needs are expressed, social engagement with family and friends and maintaining relationships can create engaging and shared joyful moments and support individuals and their family and friends.

So much money is being raised to find a "cure" for Alzheimer's disease and other causes of dementia. Walks are organized, benefit golf tournaments are popular, tribute donations are given, and even funding from the US government are all reputable efforts to find a cure or medication for cognitive decline. Unfortunately, after over three decades of research and billions of dollars, there is still no cure. Medications have been introduced to "manage the symptoms," but often, the side effects, exuberant costs, and minimal benefits, families continue to wait, hanging their hats and hoping that the "cure" is just around the corner.

Focusing on the deficits of a person with cognitive decline or any disability, the person will experience prejudices, discrimination, and isolation. The L.O.V.E Approach is a strengths-based approach, focusing on what the person can do and helps slow down the progression of the changes and create a more joyful life. The "social model" for supporting people living with cognitive decline suggests that by providing more education and awareness to society and, addressing the stigma of dementia for both the person the family, and eliminating barriers for the person being unable to truly live their full potential and a life of quality need can result in a more inclusive community.

Society and people's attitudes and misperceptions of a person diagnosed with a type of dementia are likely the biggest barriers for people living with a neurocognitive disorder to maintain a job, live more independently, and maintain autonomy with opportunities for making their own choices. The eco-psychosocial approach to wellness includes activities to promote physical, cognitive, and social health. Supporting someone living with dementia must be a "person-centered approach." Getting to know the individual as "a person" and not a "patient" and exploring the person's background, lived experiences, social history and interests while focusing on their strengths and what they are able to do rather than what they can no longer do is key.

The L.O.V.E. Approach supports this social model, and we even go beyond a "person-centered" approach and support a "family and friends-centered" approach. Staying active in the community with familiar people and familiar places and living an active and engaged life enhances the stimulation the person needs to maintain independence as long as possible.

Perhaps you have heard this story...

A little girl was helping her mother prepare dinner. Like so many times before, when her mother was preparing a roast beef dinner, she always cut the ends off the roast before placing it in the pot. The little girl had been curious about this for some time and finally asked her mother why she cut the ends off the roast before placing it in the pot. With no hesitation, her mother answered, "Because my mother did it this way." This piqued the child's curiosity, who immediately ran to her grandmother and asked her why she cut the ends off the roast before putting it in the pot and, without thinking, stated, "My mother did it this way."

The little girl continued on her quest to discover the real answer and asked her great-grandmother why she cut the ends off the roast before putting it in the pot. Her great-grandmother matter-of-factly replied, "Well honey, my pot just wasn't big enough, so I had to cut the ends off so it would fit."

I don't recall when I first heard this parable, but it has stuck with me, and I use it often to encourage people and organizations to examine long-held beliefs. I am sure there are several versions to tell, but the lesson is clear. Not questioning the reason or rationale for continuing to use the same approach because it has "always done that way" stifles creativity and opportunities to find new innovative strategies to improve upon an idea or technique.

So when it comes to treating persons living with Alzheimer's disease and other dementia, should we continue to cut the ends off our roast (interact the way we always have) or buy a bigger pot (try new strategies and communication skills)? I believe we need to buy a bigger pot and move beyond the "bio-medical model" that focuses on the neurological changes in the brain and focus on the person and their family.

Millions of dollars are poured annually into finding the cause and a cure when the answer is unknown, and that answer may not be available for many more years. So, should we shift our paradigm on how we treat people with dementia and begin to use a more eco-psychosocial approach, learning how, through engagement, we can reduce our loved ones' anxiety, depression, stress, and even apathy that some drugs actually cause as side effects?

I believe there needs to be significant changes in the approach to how we support (or don't support) people living with Alzheimer's disease and other dementias. There just needs to be more support for these families. Please don't misunderstand me. We need research, but alternative treatment approaches need to be included in those research dollars and assist individuals and families who are already impacted by dementia and have more emphasis on "living well with dementia" today.

So why are families not using this approach? One, families are not aware of the social model of treatment, and secondly, it is not as easy as dispensing a pill they think might help. The day-to-day stress that a family member can experience when caring for a loved one diagnosed with a neurocognitive disorder may feel like it is just additional work rather than understanding it is a perfect way to stay connected and can be easily done with the appropriate training. Research shows that staying engaged with the person with memory loss and participating in activities together can reduce many of the unmet needs that are presented as anxiety and worry. When someone is engaged in a meaningful activity, there is no need to exhibit stress.

Many families find that developing a meaningful daily routine early into the diagnosis will make the progression of memory loss much easier. Begin the morning at breakfast ( yes, eat together) and perhaps share a daily devotion to engage in a conversation. Take a morning walk together and plan time during the day to enjoy music, dancing and singing and enhance both of your lives.

Medications may be a little helpful in treating anxiety, but learning how to validate your family member's feelings, avoiding correcting your loved one on inaccurate facts, and allowing the person to have purpose and meaning in their life by reminiscing can also work and make for a much pleasant and less stressful day. It does require changing your approach, but these changes are not only helpful to the person living with memory loss but also a natural way for family members to take care of their own well-being and improve their quality of life.

A neurocognitive disorder is a disability, and the medical model of a disability focuses on the deficits of the person; thus, the person feels excluded and undervalued because of what they cannot do. The social model, however, suggests individuals are not the cause of their disability but rather the result of environmental barriers, prejudices, stigmas, negative attitudes and ineffective communication that limits the person.

# Paradigm Shift

A person living with and without a disability wants to experience a sense of belonging, feel accepted, and have a valued and meaningful purpose in their life. Having social relationships with friends and staying active in their community promotes a life of quality. However, social inclusion of children and adults with disabilities continues to be a challenge due to a lack of education and awareness, and even disregarding the legal rights of those with a disability can occur. Discrimination of a group of people causes prejudices and preconceived beliefs of their abilities, needs, and feelings.

So, is dementia a misunderstood disability? According to the Centers for Disease Control and Prevention: "A disability is any condition of the body or mind (impairment) that makes it more difficult for the person with the condition to do certain activities (activity limitation) and interact with the world around them (participation restrictions)." This can include disabilities that affect a person's thinking, remembering, movement, learning, communication, and social relationships.

From a legal standpoint, the Americans with Disability Act (ADA) defines a person with a disability "as a person who has a physical or mental impairment that substantially limits one or more major life activities," and the person may qualify for Social Security Disability Benefits. People living with dementia are often discriminated against in the workforce, even though the ADA makes it "unlawful to discriminate against a person based on that person's association with a person with a disability." Often, people are "forced to retire" when they disclose a diagnosis of dementia at a workplace, and accommodations to adapt the job skills are seldom even considered.

Inclusion of all people in our communities is not just a legal right, but it is the right thing to do. So why do we not recognize that a person living with dementia is actually living with a chronic disability? Could better education and understanding of what dementia is and is not help lessen the stigma that a diagnosis of dementia brings to both the person and the family?

When people are excluded from participating in everyday community life, social isolation can occur, and loneliness and lack of stimulation can have adverse outcomes. We saw the sad and serious consequences of social isolation of our seniors living alone during the COVID-19 pandemic. Keeping you and your family member active in your community, and especially in social opportunities or your church, is so important to reduce the loneliness of dementia. Staying connected with others improves overall well-being, not only for the person with dementia but also for the family and friends.

What we believe about the rules of right and wrong and our perceptions toward certain groups of people, such as the LGBTQ community, people of color, people with disabilities, mental health, racism and dementia, these perceptions affect our behaviors. These are all paradigms or perspectives and beliefs are a set of ideas or the way we look at something. Paradigms are important because they define our perspective or view of people or social issues.

So, what are your basic beliefs? Do your values match how you are actually living? How do you see the world? All of these questions help to define our personal paradigms and what guides our behaviors. A paradigm is how we look at something. Our beliefs that influence how we make decisions began with our family (parents) paradigm when we were children, often mostly influenced by our dominant parents. But as we grow up, we get more information or have a new experience and our paradigm of what we believed when we were young can change.

Several years ago, I was working with an active four-year-old boy with autism to help him improve his sensory integration and community skills. He lived near a store his mother used frequently, but Sam (not his real name) was unable to process all the sounds, lights, and smells or use words to express his fears and would either refuse to go in or scream throughout the store. This, of course, was embarrassing to his mom because these behaviors would draw attention and receive judgmental looks from strangers.

The store was within walking distance to their home, so for two months, four times a week, Sam and I would walk to the store, and at first, he exhibited the same fears that Mom described. Sam was a smart little guy, and when we first began our mission, Sam would turn and walk away from the store when we were in eyeshot. I had toys to help distract him, but he wasn't buying what I was selling! After the first month, Sam would walk to the parking lot, and we would play and return home.

Eventually, Sam entered the store through the automatic doors, quickly turned to his left and exited through the other automatic door. With patience and hard work on Sam's part, we were finally able to walk around the store with no incidents. Unlike his mom, who felt the pain of her son, a therapist doesn't have the same reactions as family members when they find themselves in an embarrassing situation due to unusual social behaviors.

On this particular day, after practicing for several weeks, Sam was prepared for the whole experience. He was ready to go shopping. He had a five-dollar bill in one hand and an empty tube of toothpaste in the other to match the tube. When the automatic doors opened, rather than looping through the exit door as he did in the beginning, he eagerly walked to the toothpaste aisle (he knew the store well!), matched the tube, and then we headed to check out. Now I need to let you know at this point that Sam was a busy little boy and enjoyed touching things. As we stood in line, Sam meticulously took his tiny index finger and began touching every candy bar, breath mint rolls, and anything else within reach.

He made little noises, and as we moved closer to the register, he was having a great time doing no harm to the items. As we took a step closer, I caught a glimpse of a woman behind us with a little boy about Sam's age, and she gave me the "look." You know the look. The judgmental, "stink eye" glance that people give when they are passing judgment on you. She thought I didn't notice, "And then." we locked eyes. Her facial expressions gave her away, and it was clear she had an issue with Sam touching the items in the impulse aisle, so accurately referred to.

She probably thought I was a horrible mother who did not teach my son appropriate "waiting in line skills," didn't enforce the "no touching rule," and felt the need to let me know nonverbally. The line was moving at a snail's pace, so I decided this mom and I needed to connect. Sam's mom was awesome, and when I asked what Sam's superpowers and purpose in life were, she proudly shared that it was to teach others about autism. Being a strong advocate and champion for the underdogs, I always take advantage of an impromptu "teachable moment" to help others understand disabilities, and Sam and I were ready to share his purpose in life.

I turned toward my new friend, smiled and calmly stated, "You know, standing in line when you are four years old can be tough." She was surprised and startled that I spoke to her and sheepishly replied, "I guess it is." Of course, her little boy was standing very still next to her like a little angel. As I made the comment, she quickly placed her hand in the center of his back and pulled him close to her leg. He was a bit startled as well but complied.

I continued my conversation and asked if she knew much about autism. She replied that she didn't, standing very stoic. I continued and shared that Sam had autism and sensory difficulties, and two months ago, he couldn't even come into the store. She began to relax a bit but still had a firm hold on her son as if to protect him from possibly catching autism. I resumed my one-sided conversation and explained the hard work Sam had done to be able to overcome his intense fear of unfamiliar sounds, bright lights and so on. She smiled, and my mission was accomplished.

Our "teachable moment" took less than a minute, and it was our turn at the register. Sam proudly placed his money and the new tube of toothpaste on the counter. The clerk smiled when she saw the satisfaction on his face, and I felt such a sense of pride for Sam.

After leaving the store, we headed to the sidewalk to return home, and I happened to look back and spotted the mother and her son as they walked to their car. But her son wasn't walking beside her. She was carrying him in her arms and holding him so tight I think I saw those perfect little angel wings pop out. I wondered if she was so grateful her son didn't have autism and perhaps understood, for the first time, the challenges and sacrifices parents must make when a child has a disability.

By experiencing an emotional interaction with me and little Sam that morning, even for a short period of time, Mom's paradigm or belief about autism possibly shifted a bit and perhaps even chipped away at the stigma she and so many others have about children like Sam. Although Sam wasn't aware of the influence he had on that mom about understanding autism a bit better, Sam's mom knew how important it was for her son to have a purpose in his life.

Much like Sam, people living with dementia may be unable to identify their life's purpose. It is, therefore, our job to help cultivate a meaningful life by focusing on their gifts, strengths, and abilities. All people need to feel useful, and people with dementia or Alzheimer's disease are no different. By cultivating a healthy sense of self for your loved one, studies show helping your loved one to feel proud, helpful, and respected and allowing them the right to maintain their dignity helps them to see themselves as valuable people and live meaningful lives. According to research, a sense of purpose in life is associated with healthier cognitive outcomes throughout adulthood, including those with dementia."

I never saw that mom or the little boy again on our walks, but my guess is she shared that experience with others and unknowingly became an advocate for children with autism. Humanizing Sam allowed her to experience an emotional interaction, and she saw that little boy differently by the end of our encounter.

As our population ages and the rate of dementia and Alzheimer's disease continues to rise, we must find alternative approaches to supporting those with dementia and their families. We cannot continue to do what we are doing "because it has always been done that way" without questioning whether there is another way. I believe we need to buy a bigger pot and begin approaching dementia differently. I hope you agree and will join me and try engaging in life with L.O.V.E.

For over four decades, I have fought the stigma attached to so many of my clients: addiction and alcoholism, mental health, autism, children and adults with developmental disabilities, Special Olympics athletes and other marginalized groups. While I will always advocate for basic human rights, inclusion, diversity and equity, I have found a special place and passion for persons living with dementia and their families, so now I fight for you.

## Activity 1

Go to your search engine, Google or another and search the word "dementia."

1. Write down your perception of the pictures and words.

2. Now return to the search engine and search "recreation and dementia." and again write down your perception.

3. Did the two different searches create any emotions or self-awareness? Write your responses below.

## Activity 2

Are you beginning to see your family member differently? Write down your response.

## Activity 3

Write down something you learned from this chapter.

## Activity 4

Identify two new ideas that you are willing to try with your loved one.

# Chapter 3
# Engaging in Life

*"I have a burning desire to live!" - A gentleman living with mixed dementia.*

When facilitating a group, I always begin by asking the participants to "Tell me something good!" In groups supporting people with dementia, the response may be as simple as "I'm here!" or "It's a great day!" But one morning, a man who had been attending one of my groups for a couple of months surprised us all when he shouted out, "I have a burning desire to live!"

At the time, the gentleman and his wife were participating in a weekly dyadic social group for people living with memory loss with a family member. The group is designed to simultaneously engage the person with dementia and a family member and enjoy a robust program addressing the social, physical, cognitive, emotional, and spiritual domains of well-being. Using a strengths-based approach to create meaningful activities, your positive interactions can allow the family members to experience the gifts and skills of their loved ones.

A dyadic group helps family members learn new strategies and skills to encourage their loved ones to become more interactive and communicate more effectively, especially for those with dementia and language difficulties. Through the staff's modeling of communication and engagement techniques during the group, this method strengthens the possibility that these skills will have carry-over value at home.

When the gentleman began attending the group, he would occasionally comment about his frustrations with his memory loss. His affect was flat, and his wife was speaking for him and correcting him frequently. After a few months into the program, she told me that learning how to communicate, giving him choices, and breaking up tasks into smaller chunks were a game changer for them.

During the first month of the couple's participation in the group, this gentleman's mood improved, and it was apparent he was enjoying the socialization as he began arriving with a smile and a handshake and would leave with a heartfelt promise to "See you next week." His wife reported they both looked forward to the group. She was more positive and encouraged at home and had established a routine with a morning reading and a walk. As she was learning ways to incorporate meaning into his day and sharing common interests, they were having fewer conflicts. Not only were her beliefs shifting about dementia, but he too began to change the way he saw himself.

Practicing patience and new communication skills was difficult for her in the beginning, but as she began empowering him to do more for himself, she discovered the importance for her husband to maintain his independence, even if it took longer to complete daily living tasks.

Encouraging the families to continue participating in activities they have enjoyed in the past is so important for quality of life. This couple learned to live life to the fullest, enjoying the simple pleasure of their day. They began to visit the museums they once loved and renewed their annual theatre tickets. By seeking experiences that brought them joy and happiness, they continued to make beautiful memories together. She became a pro at adapting their activities and keeping them both engaged in life as his cognitive decline progressed.

The far-reaching health benefits of staying active can influence how we see ourselves and how others see us. Our efforts give purpose to our days and by contributing to your community, you can bring more meaning to your life. It is unfortunate that so many families isolate and withdraw from the world rather than learn how to live well with dementia.

Each new skill set I developed throughout my career helped form the foundation of the L.O.V.E Approach for individuals, their families and friends living with a neurocognitive disorder. The uniqueness of this approach focuses on helping family and friends change how they speak to their family members and how to resolve unfamiliar situations (teach to fish) rather than just providing the answer (give a fish). Each person is different, and there is no standard answer to most situations that may arise.

*"Give a man a fish and you feed him for a day. Teach him how to fish and you feed him for a lifetime"* Chinese philosopher Lao Tzu.

By implementing the L.O.V.E. Approach, you learn how to identify your family member's needs that trigger a concerning behavior and better understand how your family member communicates through their behaviors. All behaviors have a purpose, and by listening, observing, validating, and engaging with your friend or family member, you will learn how to adapt when neurological changes occur and be better prepared for the future.

As mentioned earlier, self-efficacy training for family and friends, in-depth understanding of the dementia-related behavioral symptoms, a shift in beliefs about people living with dementia, advocation for the person, self-care, and utilizing effective psychosocial interventions, family members and friends can have a more positive experience while supporting the family member at home. **A supportive relationship with family members or friends is essential when considering the health outcomes in the home environment.**

The L.O.V.E Approach is based on that same methodology, giving you, your family or your friend the tools to feel capable, confident, and informed to practice effective communication strategies and maintain connectedness and engagement by developing the skills necessary to become a more creative problem solver and confident decision maker. Positive outcomes are also determined by the satisfaction, rewards, and personal growth of the family members and the person living with memory loss.

My work has always been a spiritual path. Pat Head's diagnosis of early-onset Alzheimer's disease was the pivotal moment when I was called to gain an in-depth understanding of dementia and the impact it has on families. I trained to be a Certified Dementia Practitioner (CDP) in the winter of 2011, the year of Pat's diagnosis, and the next chapter of my life began.

I have always heard that good ideas are not complex. Sue Grafton, a favorite mystery writer of mine, once said, "Ideas are easy. It's the executive that really separates the sheep from the goats." The L.O.V.E. Approach consists of four simple concepts that may seem difficult to master in the beginning, but with practice and the guidance and coaching you will find in this book, you will begin to believe you can learn the skills you need to begin sharing joyful moments again.

The common thread that runs through the four concepts of the L.O.V.E. approach: listening, observing, validating, and engaging is learning and practicing effective communication skills. So, borrowing from a popular song from the late "Queen of Rock 'n' Roll," Tina Turner, you may ask, *What's Love Got to Do With It?*

Loving someone with any form of dementia can be complicated and heartbreaking at the same time. Often, the neurological progression can present changes in the person's personality and perception of reality, causing confusion for both of you. A father, for example, may think his daughter is his wife because, in his mind, he may be quite young, and the daughter may look like her mother during that time.

Time shifting usually occurs in the later progression of neurological changes, and the person thinks it is an earlier time in their life. When the person can no longer keep track of time or know the days of the week or even the seasons, being able to know when they had a meal or a visit from the grandchildren becomes impossible.

People living with dementia may forget your name and who you are, but they always remember how you make them feel. I worked with a woman for over three years, and during that time, she identified her superpower as "Living this long." She was ninety-three at the time. As her needs changed, her son and daughter-in-law loved her so much that they realized they could no longer provide the support she needed at home. She transitioned into a memory care community near their home, and family and beloved dog visit regularly.

I provided coaching along the way, suggesting questions to ask the communities when making a choice, learning how to advocate for their family member, and even tips on moving furniture and personal belongings to her new home. I still visit her occasionally and she does not remember who I am or how our lives crossed, but she always smiles and pats the chair next to her, calls me "Honey," and invites me "To come sit down." While we sit, she places her hand on my forearm and we watch the birds and squirrels out the big picture window, and sometimes we sing her favorite hymns.

There are many forms of love and it usually refers to the feeling between two people. I won't attempt to go into the deep philosophical definition of love but just point out that love can be expressed in many different ways. Whether it is family love or the love of a friend, we all need to feel loved and to give love. We also need to feel we belong somewhere, feel special and valued with a sense of autonomy and make our own decisions as long as possible.

With the progression of dementia, the increase of vulnerability and dependence on others does as well. The reasons friends or family members decide to accept the responsibility of providing care for someone with dementia in the home vary. A study done in 2019 identified four categories of motivation: moral-based motives, religious and spiritual motives, financial motives, and "wicked" motives such as the possibility of inheriting the house or access to their financial information or the possibility of inheriting large sums of money at the person's death. (6)

I have to believe that most people make the commitment to care for the person out of love and not just obligation. Even if you were not close to the person prior to the dementia diagnosis, providing support offers an opportunity to resolve negative feelings, and your relationship may possibly become stronger. Focusing on what is really important to you can also give you a sense of purpose and result in a deeper connection to your loved one or friend.

Once you decide to become a primary support person for a friend or loved one with dementia, you make a commitment with many consequential responsibilities and the acceptance that you will make many sacrifices. Your life will change and the care you provide will determine the person's health outcomes and well-being. Taking care of your own healthcare needs is crucial in order to provide the support a person with dementia may require.

If you ensure the person's autonomy, or having the capacity to make choices and decisions about their care, remain as independent as possible, and stay engaged in life, the person can thrive, and the progression of cognitive decline will slow. There may come a point when the person can no longer make an informed decision, but until then, encouraging the person to decide what they want to wear, eat, or do is their right. On the other hand, if you accept the responsibility to care for your loved one and choose not to provide this level of care, the person's cognitive loss will decline faster.

You are also responsible for the person receiving the medical care they need, providing proper supervision to maintain their safety, offering nutritious meals, providing assistance with activities of daily living, and creating opportunities for socialization and enjoying the outdoors. People with dementia have rights, just as anyone does, and the person must be respected when you commit to being the person they trust the most.

People living with dementia have the right to be treated as adults and spoken to with respect. They should be given the opportunity to experience meaningful activities throughout the day. When a family commits to providing 24-hour support, the family should receive the proper training necessary to communicate and engage with the person so he/she can continue to feel purpose, enjoy a life of quality, and maintain relationships. Having a purpose in life directly relates to better physical and emotional health and can help decrease stress for both the person and the family member.

If these key responsibilities are neglected, your loved one is at risk for falls, malnutrition, getting lost by leaving the house unsupervised, weight loss, depression from loneliness and isolation, poor hygiene, and emergency room visits. Even when you choose to support the person out of love, there may be times when you become frustrated, overwhelmed and even angry with your loved one. There is nothing wrong with having feelings. However, it is imperative to learn how to regulate your emotions and not react to the concerning behaviors of your loved one.

Staying socially active and engaged with friends and family members relieves stress, boosts self-esteem, and alleviates the boredom, isolation, and loneliness that people with dementia often experience. Social interaction is healthy and can slow symptoms of dementia, including cognitive functioning and memory loss.

Providing a high level of support is possible when caring for someone at home, but you must be willing to make sacrifices and learn how to engage with your loved one. If there comes a time when this is no longer possible, finding an alternative living arrangement is the best and fairest decision you can make for the person you love. I caution families not to agree with a person to "Never put me in a home" but rather promise them you will always take care of them and love them. This helps with the guilt the family feels and prevents so many people with dementia from living in an unhealthy environment, when in reality, deciding and asking for help is the kindest and loving gesture you can make.

*"Love life. Engage in it. Give it all you've got. Love it with a passion because life truly does give back, many times over, what you put into it."* — Maya Angelou.

# Activity 1

## Purpose in Life

1. What is your purpose in life? What is the meaning of your life?

2. Ask your loved one his/her purpose in life. Get input and assist the person in identifying his/her contribution to things that are meaningful and important.

# Activity 2

## Identifying Your Skill Sets

List the skill sets that are or can be useful to support your loved one. (Organizational skills, listening skills, coping skills)

# Activity 3

## Identifying Your Circle of Support

1. Make a list of family members, friends, church members, or neighbors you can call on for support. (Pick up milk at the grocery, stop by and have coffee, just talk.)

2. Add people to your list:

3. Identify the people with whom you have not shared the diagnosis/circumstance but know you need to. (I know it's hard!)

4. Identify one person from the above question and reach out. (You can do this!)

## Chapter 4
## The L.O.V.E. Approach:
## Listen, Observe, Validate, and Engage

**Listen**

Several years ago, I was managing a summer camp in San Francisco and was meeting with a young boy on the autism spectrum and his mom. He was excited to be coming to camp for the first time, and I needed to understand how he best communicated his needs, learn his interests, and identify his strengths so he would have a fun and successful summer.

His mother was sitting with us at the table when he suddenly jumped out of his chair, placed his hands firmly over both ears and began jumping around. It is not unusual for a child or an adult with autism to have hypersensitivity to sounds, but I heard nothing. I looked to his mom to understand the cause of this abrupt change in her son, and she placed two fingers to her lips to communicate we should remain quiet, then whispered one word to me: "Listen." So, with our eyes locked, we listened with great effort and could barely hear the faint hum of a lawn mower in the very far distance. Mom just smiled proudly at me, possibly for her child's remarkable gift.

His mother reported that he hears noises before others can, and some sounds, such as a lawnmower, are painful to his ears. But unlike people living with dementia, who may have lost their abilities to problem solve or use strategies from the past to manage emotions and feelings that can cause stress, this little boy knew how to let us know he was beginning to feel something painful and protected himself by covering both ears.

This little boy taught me the importance of listening when supporting someone living with dementia. It is our responsibility to practice active listening for the sounds and the silences, and by being proactive, we can avert possible stressful events and help our family members living with dementia feel safe. Identifying noises in your home, such as the hum or absence of the hum of an air conditioner, can be troubling. Barking dogs, background noise from the television, dishes clanging as you load the dishwasher, a vacuum cleaner, a doorbell, and, like the little boy, a lawnmower may trigger an unexpected attempt for your loved one to communicate a need.

Like young Sam, who could not process the auditory and visual stimulus in his neighborhood store, noises in the community will need to be assessed as well. Horns honking, sirens, trains, or loud people in a restaurant can trigger a stressful situation, and unlike the little boy who knew to cover his ears, coping skills for people with dementia have diminished, and they are unable to understand or regulate their emotions. Thus, they may use body language, sudden movements, or a shrill to communicate their discomfort. All behaviors have a purpose, and by learning to observe and listen, you can help your family member or friend manage their stress and anxiety and feel physically and emotionally safe.

Actively listening not only includes listening for unpleasant noises that may irritate or startle your loved one but also taking the time to really listen to understand without responding when practicing new ways to communicate. Language difficulties are common with dementia, and giving the person time to really listen to the words (or lack of words, such as body language) will make communication easier. When people don't take the time to listen and understand, the person with dementia feels misunderstood, and conflicts occur. Listening to the person, not the dementia, is important to understand, and by accepting their reality, you can join them where they are.

My dad would often tell me I was given "Two ears and one mouth and should listen more than I talk." I am sure my father was not quoting the great Greek philosopher Epictetus when he shared this wisdom, but they are both correct. Listening is not about hearing but rather about focused attention when listening.

It wasn't long ago before a friend and her family were visiting a wildlife park in Florida and attended a presentation on the manatee. The guide was very enthusiastic and was positioned in front of a row of bleachers overlooking the park's observatory. My friend's young niece was very attentive, taking in every word.

At the end of the presentation, the guide invited questions. The little girl quickly popped up her arm and waved her small hand as her parents gleamed with pride for their daughter's inquisitive nature. She waited patiently, and when she was finally called on, she pointed her two little feet toward the guide, wiggled her stubby little toes and responded with her own profound question. "Do you like my new sandals?"

When we have our own agenda and are busy thinking about our next comment rather than "listening," we miss the emotion behind what is being said. Learning a new skill takes practice. Enhancing your communication skills to better interact with a person having difficulty processing information also takes practice and patience, but it is well worth the effort as interactions will become more pleasant and meaningful and reduce stress for everyone. By gaining a greater awareness of how we talk and listen, relationships become more meaningful, and connections become stronger.

One of the worst things we can do to destroy a healthy relationship is to point out mistakes and correct a person. Correcting someone with dementia is particularly harmful as they feel shame and embarrassment often over an insignificant fact or detail. So why do people constantly correct someone?

Often, the "corrector" may be a "black and white thinker" or have a natural way of believing that everything is either "right or wrong." Being able to let go of simple mistakes that don't quite fit their ideas is difficult and upsetting. This causes resentment from the person constantly being corrected. Unwavering attempts to insist someone with dementia recall a fact or point out "wrong" or incorrect statements create feelings of inadequacy, and the person will eventually stop trying. Apparently, some people are just pedantic, letting nothing inaccurate get by.

Correcting the person living with memory loss most often results in an argument. This is upsetting and makes them angry and will create a situation that could easily be avoided. Please note: You will never win an argument with a person with dementia! Being corrected also may result in the person living with dementia feeling they are being treated like a "child." This can also cause resentment and motivation to not share feelings or thoughts or even complete tasks. This will also quickly erode the trust in a relationship. If a fact or memory is incorrect, it really shouldn't matter. It is your issue, not theirs.

Avoid asking a person who cannot remember to remember. Asking a person living with short-term memory loss what they had for breakfast is pointless. The memory of breakfast cannot be stored because of the changes in the brain thus the person cannot retrieve the memory. Avoid continually correcting a person living with memory loss when they believe a deceased loved one is still living. Often, people with dementia expect their mother for lunch, who died many years ago.

Rather than reminding your loved one that his/her mother had died, encourage the person to talk about their mother and recall joyful memories they shared, such as favorite foods or places that they visited together. They will relive the sad news that their mom is deceased every time you tell them. Each time you tell them about the death, it will be as if it is the first time they hear it every single time.

Also, take the blame rather than shame a person living in their altered reality. When the person is angry that the car keys are not where they had left them, even though they have not driven for years, blame yourself for misplacing them and assure your loved one that you will look for them. He may think he needs something from the store, and he is trying to meet that need. Explore what he might be seeking, as it could be possible he is just hungry. Taking time to really listen and understand takes practice, but once you are able to not just hear but feel what the person is sharing, connections grow stronger.

I usually get pushback when I give this suggestion because we are programmed to automatically jump into a fight or flight mode when we experience criticism. This may not be an imperfection in our personalities; it's just our brain protecting us.

I recall so vividly the shame and embarrassment a man experienced during an assessment with me regarding his memory loss. His wife had reached out about a year prior to the assessment, and we had spoken several times throughout the year. She finally made an appointment to attend a social group. Sadly, it is not uncommon for families to avoid seeking help in the earlier stages of dementia due to denial or the stigma felt. Couples tend to want to "take care of it themselves" and are hesitant to even ask for help from their family.

Common reasons parents do not want to call on their children is because "my son has his own life" or "my daughter already has her hands full with the grandchildren." It has been my experience that once adult children realize how much help is really needed, they are hurt that they were not told the truth about the situation and the severity of the dementia.

When the gentleman and his wife finally came to the appointment, I greeted them both with a handshake and a smile and introduced myself. Whenever I begin to engage with someone, I always "get on their train" by finding a common thread or interest with the person. This is helpful in creating a trusting relationship. As we walked to my office, I noticed he was wearing a Marine Corps hat and decided that was going to be my "in" to get on his train.

Once seated, the man hung his head and placed his hands in his lap as if he had been called into the principal's office. I jumped right in and told the man I had noticed his Marine Corps hat and shared that my father was a Marine, and he had always told me, "Once a Marine, always a Marine." The man immediately raised his head, turned toward me and looked straight into my eyes. He removed his hat with purpose and proudly pointed to the familiar "Semper Fi" motto on the brim of his cap. Latin for "Always faithful," this motto signifies the loyalty and bond between every Marine. When given the opportunity, I always thank veterans for their service, and when I expressed my gratitude to this proud Marine, it opened the door for him to walk through and tell me his story. As he recalled memories of his service years, he transformed from a man struggling with memory and confusion to the honorable Marine he was over fifty years ago.

We continued to chat and he became more animated and enthusiastic about his younger days and even reached and gently touched my arm as a gesture we were connected. More than likely, his wife had heard this story many times, and she sat quietly by his side until he told me he was discharged after the war in 1986. It was obvious to me what year he was thinking, so I ignored the date and let him continue. However, his wife suddenly interrupted to correct him. "Honey, it was 1946, not 1986," she stated matter-of-factly. As quickly as we connected and this gentleman felt safe to tell me his story earlier, the shame and humiliation occurred just as fast. I am sure you have seen the shame I speak of.

Because she pointed out his mistake, he was embarrassed, and his conversation with me, a new friend, suddenly ended. He dropped his head and reverted back to a sad, timid, meek man with dementia I had only met twenty minutes ago, and he completely shut down. It took several minutes for him to speak again, but I could see in his eyes that he continued to feel shame. Persons with dementia can continue to feel shame even after they forget what caused it.

Think of a time you felt embarrassed or shamed for a mistake someone pointed out. Perhaps you mispronounced a word, or you got caught in a little white lie. Feelings of being exposed to our mistakes affect our self-esteem and self-worth. Repeatedly feeling shame can cause a person to lose belief and faith in the "constant corrector" and can be at high risk of developing depression and anxiety.

As memories disappear, people with dementia repeat stories from their past. The person can recall long-term memories (although not always accurately) as those memories have been stored for thirty or forty years, or like the proud Marine, for over fifty years. Because short-term memory loss affects the brain's ability to store new memories, stories and questions are repeated again and again as the person is unable to remember what they just talked about. Believe me, they are not doing this is annoy you, but perhaps only seeking interaction, conversation and a feeling of connectedness. Feelings of loneliness and boredom are two of the most common complaints from people who live with dementia, so encouraging your loved one to share stories from their past can alleviate both of these feelings.

Friends are so often kept in the dark when a friend is diagnosed with dementia. Friends really want to know how to support their friend living with a neurocognitive disorder. They miss their friend and feel left out of the person's life and confused. A friend of mine had a dear golfing buddy who developed dementia. My friend tried taking her golfing but was frustrated her friend was not holding the club correctly or understanding the game any longer. When we explored ways they could continue this activity, their golf outings became fun again.

My friend was able to change her expectations of what golf is and adjust to her friend's reality. She realized it was their friendship that really mattered, not golf. They would go to the course and ride around in a golf cart and were able to continue to find joy in their shared interest. Research shows that golf is a skill that will stay with a person with cognitive decline the longest, possibly due to the outdoor environment, socializing at the club and muscle memory.

Another good friend of mine is a golf professional teaching lessons in an active senior living community. She recognizes some golfers experience confusion and memory loss, forgetting a tee time or showing up two hours early or without their clubs. She graciously accommodates the person as she is determined to keep golfers involved in the sport they love for as long as possible. I have great admiration for her, not just as a friend but as an advocate for people living with dementia and their family members. She is doing what so many other golf professionals could do, serving these families whose quality of life could greatly improve with simple adaptations.

The L.O.V.E Approach invites friends to be involved in supporting someone with dementia from the beginning of the diagnosis. Friends often are the first to notice the changes in a person experiencing memory loss and confusion but are reluctant to say anything to the family. They may fear their own vulnerability to developing a neurocognitive disorder and may not want to watch their friend change.

However, friends are important in a dementia journey as they can provide encouragement and help the person maintain a social identity. I recently had a gentleman reach out about his friend, who he noticed was having memory lapses and difficulty finding words. He was not sure what to do. Unbeknown to him, other friends had noticed it as well, and by sheer chance, the friends ran into each other and didn't know they had all noticed the same changes in their friend, and they began to visit with their friend regularly.

*"The word 'listen' contains the same letters as the word 'silent' -Alfred Brende.*

## Observe

*"You can observe a lot by just watching."*
*-Yogi Berra*

Along with developing active listening skills, observation skills are necessary to practice your awareness of all five senses so you can recognize, understand and process your loved one's environment. By becoming more skilled at mindfulness and staying present, you will learn to become aware of your emotions and to able to use empathy and compassion to communicate effectively.

Observing your family members' emotions, reactions, and body language is crucial, as well as being able to identify and regulate your own emotions. This will improve your relationships, ensure more meaningful connections and positive interactions, and create more self-awareness. This promotes personal growth and better decision-making skills for you that will be helpful in all aspects of your life.

Keeping a journal of your observations can be helpful to look back and recognize the timeline of changes and perhaps help with future planning. Another journal that is helpful to start is a gratitude journal. Research shows that people who write down something they are thankful for each day are happier people.

Gaining insight into your own body language and how it is interpreted by your family member or friend will become easier with practice. Observing facial expressions, body language, and tone of voice and focusing on their emotional response will let you know if they are feeling understood and validated. Effective communication skill helps you connect with your family member and build meaningful relationships. When you are able to recognize your family members' emotional state, you can adjust your emotions and communicate without conflict easier. All behaviors are communication, and we must understand what behavior is telling us.

If we ask someone with dementia to do something and they refuse, we can honor their choice rather than characterizing the person as "non-cooperative." Negative social-emotional responses can result in a person with dementia feeling judged, devalued and emotionally unsafe. By using a strength-based approach to support, you will recognize what the person is capable of and what they have to offer.

Sherlock Holmes, the fictional British "consulting detective," had uncanny observation skills and a knack for deductive reasoning. His success came from his amazing senses and persistence to not give up. Jessica Fletcher, on the other hand, was a fictional mystery writer who lived in Cabot Cove, a fictional coastal town that possibly had the highest murder rate in the United States. She used her homespun charm to connect with others, often even with the murderer, and could observe the smallest details.

Although styles differed in Holmes and Fletcher to solve a crime, they both used their observation skills to assess their surroundings and take note of any unusual circumstance attentively and intentionally. With practice, sharpening your mind to take in and interpret information can eventually become a helpful habit.

Having worked in clinical settings half of my career, it was necessary to be able to enter a room and quickly identify any patterns of behavior that might need to be immediately addressed, recognize changes or symptoms in a client's health condition, determine any safety risk factors in the environment, and to be able to prioritize and develop a strategy to resolve any concerns quickly.

Notice the changes around you and minimize distractions. Is the television on throughout the day, or should you schedule your lawn care to come at a better time? Is there too much stimulus in sight, such as too many clothes in the closet, making it difficult for the person to select from?

Are summer and winter clothes still in the closet, making decisions even more confusing? One of the early signs of cognitive changes is a person wearing inappropriate clothing for a season or the weather conditions. Recognizing the need to change dirty clothes can also be difficult for someone with dementia. If the person has agnosia and is unable to process sensory information, they may not see the stains or smell the dirty clothes. If you leave the person's "favorite" dirty clothes in a hamper and do not wash them right away, the person may see the clothes, which can trigger the person to redress with the dirty clothes, so keeping dirty clothes out of sight is best. Your family member needs to have choices in what they wear, especially around the house, but limiting the choices may make it easier for him/her to make decisions.

Check the floor and look for things that can lead to a fall. Should a rug be stored to lower the risk of the person tripping or getting a walker hung up on the edge? Go room to room and identify safety concerns and remove or store items that may be dangerous. Make sure certain knives, scissors, and other dangerous items, such as chemicals, are locked away.

Keep valuables and other important items such as jewelry, medications, keys, cell phones, and money in one place and out of sight and reach of the person. Choosing a room in the house that can be locked is a great way to keep important personal items safe. Seeing keys and money may trigger the person to leave the house and "go to the store."

Chances are you are rushing around all day trying got get tasks completed, meals prepared, and tend to household responsibilities. Slowing down may not feel like an option, but finding a place to train your brain to observe your surroundings with more attention and focus will not only provide a calmer environment, but you will also be able to use strategies to do things for yourself and have a more positive outlook.

Activating your superpowers during difficult times to problem solve, adjust to any neurological changes in your family member, or handle stressors related to your own health can empower you to tackle new challenges. Using your internal powers to address external challenges is possible when you cut out the distractions and are open to new ways of thinking. Is your superpower kindness? Perseverance? Patience? Courage? Being open-minded? Forgiveness or humor? By tapping into your character strengths, you can focus and improve your decision-making and problem-solving skills.

Knowing and understanding the specific neurocognitive disorder your loved one has is necessary for recognizing how to support your loved one. That is only one reason why a proper diagnosis is confirmed. Living with some type of dementia not only affects the person's memory but also interferes with the person's ability to process information, organize thoughts, and demonstrate logical thinking. Those challenges can lead to repetitive and concerning behaviors.

One troubling behavior is when objects go missing. This causes frustration for family members, who often confuse hiding objects in the house as hoarding. However, hoarding is a true disorder and may be a symptom of obsessive-compulsive disorder or a compulsive shopping disorder and is unrelated to dementia or Alzheimer's disease. Having the inability to throw away possessions and having overwhelming feelings of embarrassment about all the "possessions" is symptomatic of hoarding disorder.

Hiding objects by a person living with memory loss is a coping mechanism to make some sense of the confusing world they now live in or an attempt to try to gain some control over their situation. A morning muffin may be found days later under a bed pillow only because the person may have wanted a late-night snack, then, of course, forgets the muffin. Delusional thinking can be a characteristic of dementia and may cause a person to think that others are stealing from them; thus, they have the need to hide certain belongings.

There is logical reason in the person's mind when hiding the object, but because of dementia, it makes little sense to us. Be mindful that hiding objects has some purpose for the individual, and scolding is tempting, but showing patience, understanding, and empathy is important.

Paying attention to items that may "disappear" or be out of place will help you understand more about the thought process of your loved one. For instance, someone who works in an office may find and hide familiar objects such as pens, papers, mail, stamps, checkbooks, and other office supplies in an attempt to fulfill a need to be useful or go to work. The person may even see this as an effort to put all the supplies in a safe place and "help" organize the house.

If the person begins to look for a specific item, help them look, then suggest a coffee break and assure them you will help look later. They will forget the item, and this will minimize their anxiety and yours as well. Always check trash containers before taking them out or hide all trash containers, as this is a common place to put objects that the person deems unnecessary.

A person living with memory loss makes every effort in their power to be useful, have a purpose, and have meaning in their life through their behaviors. Although the behaviors are troublesome and even dangerous at times, it is your responsibility to ensure a safe and secure home environment.

Observations can be very helpful with problem-solving, and often solutions are simple. I was consulting for an assisted living community and was called to address "a behavioral problem," similar to the time the group home called about a man with Down syndrome who kept misplacing his wallet and was eventually diagnosed with dementia.

Staff were having difficulty with a new resident to shower. He did not want to walk in the shower and would stand in a waiting area or walk away. He could not verbalize why he would not shower and the staff had tried many times and continued to be unsuccessful. When I arrived at the facility, his family happened to be visiting. I introduced myself and inquired about his showering routine at home. Routines are predictable and something we can trust. His wife informed me he would shave first and then get in the shower to wash off the shaving cream.

She also told me he would always shower in the mornings before work. The staff had neglected to learn the man's bathing routine and was trying to change a forty-five-year habit to fit their agenda. When I suggested the staff reverse his shower routine and let him shave first, they gladly did. The man was satisfied and the concern was resolved. He adapted to an evening shower once the staff honored his routine.

Having routines is just a convenient way to get things done. They provide a structure that helps us manage stress and creates a more orderly life. People with dementia are able to navigate their world much better with routines. Those routines are stored in long-term memory, and since people with neurocognitive disorders have difficulty with new learning, keeping a routine helps with confusion and can reduce anxiety.

Another time, I was called in for a consultation at a memory care community. Dinner was scheduled for 5:00 p.m. each evening, and when the staff brought the residents to the dining hall, one gentleman would walk past his assigned seat, head down the hallway, and stare out a window. This was another situation where the man was unable to verbalize his needs. He would return to the dining hall at 5:20 p.m. on his own. This was troublesome to the staff as they had to reheat his meal.

I arrived at the facility at 4:45 p.m. one evening to observe this "behavior." Promptly at 5:00 p.m., staff escorted the residents to the dining room, and just like clockwork, one gentleman headed to the nearby hallway. I waited for him to get to the end of the hall, positioned at the window, and then headed down to speak to him. When I approached him, I remarked, "What a great view." I noticed he was wearing bibbed overalls and a plaid shirt. "So what are you doing?" I asked in my friendliest voice. He spoke to me without a glance and said, matter-of-fact, "Watchin' the cows come home." And sure enough, when I looked out at the large pasture, I saw perhaps 20 or 30 cows heading to a barn in the distance.

I met with the staff and recommended an accommodation by inviting a friend to dine with him around 5:20 p.m. each evening (and possibly watch the cows with him) so he could continue to enjoy something that he had possibly done most of his life. When we stop seeing these concerns as "problem behaviors" and look at them as a means of communication, solutions may be pretty simple.

## Validate

*"If you can no longer validate yourself, perhaps someone will do it for you." Vp.*

It just feels good to be validated. When your thoughts and emotions are validated by others, especially by those you love and trust, there is a feeling of acceptance and a sense of belonging. People need to feel understood, and when our feelings or thoughts are discounted or we feel misunderstood, a sudden need to stand up for ourselves is a natural response. No one likes to be invalidated.

Being able to use self-validation is important throughout our lives to help us acknowledge our strengths, abilities and talents. We use self-validation to encourage ourselves and treat ourselves with kindness, but people living with dementia may no longer be able to give themselves "pep talks" or recognize their strengths. So often, they are not validated for their feelings or ideas but rather corrected and often told how they should feel. Validation means more than just agreeing with someone about a feeling or idea; validation runs deeper and is an emotional connection with the person. Emotional validation involves expressing acceptance of another person's emotional experience.

We learn self-talk early in our childhood. Children use self-talk when learning a new skill. Watching a young child recently, I heard her reinforce her new skill when building with legos; "This one goes on top!" I was always impressed by how often Special Olympic Athletes with Down syndrome would engage in self-validation through self-talk (an out-loud conversation to one's self) to muster the motivation and courage to compete in big events. I would hear affirmations such as "I've got this" or "You can do this" as they were preparing for the event. The self-talk may have been done in private or just prior to the competition and was also used in a new social setting. Research shows that individuals with Down syndrome use self-talk as a way to cope with uncomfortable or stressful situations. Personally, I use self-talk myself at times, and not just internally. I enjoy giving myself pep talks occasionally.

Validating someone's feelings requires compassion and empathy and is not always easy. Have you ever tried to share a difficult day with someone, and rather than the person listening with compassion and concern, they responded by telling you how you could have handled it differently? Or perhaps you recognize this characteristic in yourself?

Much like the little girl who was so determined to gain affirmation from the park guide in the wildlife park, she needed to let others know how proud she was of her new sandals. The guide, by the way, did express his appreciation for her new shoes and thanked her for sharing.

Research shows that sharing stories can bring people closer together, even if they think the story is embellished. How much fun is it to be "holding court," with eyes all on you, as you share a funny or touching memory with others? Details may not match up, but does it really matter when someone is sharing a cherished memory?

I love to tell the story of the time I was attacked by a bird. My friend and I had just left Australia after snorkeling the Great Barrier Reef and were on a walking tour exploring the beautiful countryside of New Zealand. Our group had stopped at the peek of a mountain for a tea break. It was a sunny but cool morning, and while I was standing enjoying the stunning scenery, I was holding a cheese scone in my right hand and a cup of hot English breakfast tea on my left.

I was taking a sip of my tea, so my left elbow was bent and horizontally extended and apparently made for the perfect perch. Suddenly, I heard wings flapping and felt the motion of a bird directly beside my ear, and sure enough, a giant bird landed on my left forearm. I watched the bird peck the middle of my scone as if in slow motion, and tiny pieces of my breakfast biscuit levitated into the air and scatted like little snowflakes. I was so startled I fell backward, pouring the hot tea on my chest and landing on a rock, tearing my left rotor cuff.

I was certain it was a Great Australian Gannet, a large black and white bird that is widespread across the coast of the island. But my friend, with deep regret, informed me it was just a hungry little seagull. Through the years of telling my story, the bird grew much bigger, and my fall was much more dramatic. But my friend never corrected or suggested to my audience that I was embellishing or telling anything but the truth. She cared enough for me and had such compassion and grace. She had no need to correct the facts of my remarkable escapade.

This story is meaningful to me, as my friend has since passed away, and this was our last great adventure. Because of her amazing ability to show me such emotional validation, I can smile when I think of our trip. Meaningful memories and stories are meant to be told, regardless of how accurate.

Validating body language is important. Observing body language and attaching a word to what you see will help you read the message they are sending, and you can then validate by asking how they feel. Are their eyes dilated? This can often suggest a pleasant thought and a slight raise in the brows, and a slight smile may indicate confidence.

Pay attention to changes in other facial features, such as the mouth. Is their mouth beginning to tense up, or is it relaxed? Be attentive to their tone and perhaps suggest, "It looks like you are getting upset. Can I help?" Never tell another person how they feel, but only state, "It looks like," and they can deny or agree. Recognizing changes in mood and disposition will assist in being proactive and perhaps head off a distressing incident.

Delusions and hallucinations can occur in people with a neurocognitive disorder and can be effectively addressed by not overreacting. Most times, delusions and false beliefs or hallucinations are disturbing for the person with dementia. It is necessary to remain calm and validate the feeling. Often, the delusions involve people in the house or outside or some conspiracy against the person.

Responding to the underlying feelings such as fear and avoid the content of the delusion. Using validation may sound like, "That must feel really scary." Feelings are the outcome of emotion, and creating a safe place to explore the feelings of your loved one can go a long way to ensuring your loved one feels safe.

The more you learn and practice strategies to understand your loved ones, you become their best treatment. Remember, medication only treats the symptoms of dementia; you treat your loved one with a person-centered approach. Using empathy, compassion, and patience, keeping your loved one engaged in life as long as possible is the goal.

Often, assumptions are made without fully observing a movement or the way your loved my be acting. Some family members tell me they have to ask their loved ones where they are going each time they get up from the couch. I asked why they felt the need to ask, and the responses included, "I need to know where he/she is at all times," "I am afraid he/she won't find the bathroom," or "I never know what he/she will get into."

Respecting the rights of a person with dementia to have opportunities for movement, rights for privacy and dignity and access to a safe, calm environment is important. Overreacting and jumping to conclusions too quickly and result in conflicts. Observe the action, and if it is not dangerous, then let it be. If you are concerned, continue to observe if they leave the room, but discreetly as you can. Supporting your family member in the least restrictive environment can help your family member "feel at home."

Providing a safe environment and honoring the right to autonomy for a loved one with dementia requires the right balance. Being cautious is necessary, and the fear of being blamed if something should happen is always a concern for family members and causes more stress. But as you become more comfortable with your observation skills, the use of the practical skills and knowledge you have gained, providing emotional and physical support for your loved one will become more natural.

## Engage

*"Surround yourself with what you love, whether it's family, pets, keepsakes, music, plants, hobbies, whatever." – George Carlin.*

I have used the phrase "to engage" several times in earlier chapters when referring to strategies to encourage a loved one or friend living with dementia to participate in conversations, activities, and even storytelling. I have mentioned engagement can improve the person's mood, create positive feelings, improve overall well-being and enhance the quality of life for both the person and you. But how do you do this?

Meaningful engagement is a person-centered approach that invites people to participate in a "purposeful activity" that is meaningful to a person. Activities we enjoy align with our life values, ability levels, talents, gifts, and interests, such as our hobbies, volunteer work, recreational activities, sports, and even our vocation. The National Library of Medicine published a study that indicated individuals who engaged in activities more frequently had "better psychological and physical functioning."

Studies also show the positive health outcomes from remaining active and social as we age; lower blood pressure, less depression, helps manage weight, reduces risk of ideas and improves you to do the things you love. (7)

Much like emotional validation, emotional engagement also requires compassion, empathy, and an expression of acceptance for other experiences. Having a purpose in life is essential, and engaging in activities can do this. Research shows that having a purpose is important for a feeling of well-being. During the pandemic, I facilitated a weekly online social group for individuals with dementia and a family member and we were having a group on the benefits of volunteering. The family of one participant was making masks to donate, and although the woman with memory loss had not used a sewing machine for several years, her family encouraged her to try. Her muscle memory kicked in, and the mask-making project was a great success. The family saw a difference in her mood, as she suddenly had a sense of purpose using a skill she had known since making clothes for her children. Be creative when looking for opportunities for your family members to feel they can still contribute to their family or their community using their gifts and talents. Helping others can give meaning and purpose to anyone's life. When we can help a person with dementia feel heard, understood, and validated, a sense of safety and trust will lead to a social-emotional connection, and once this connection is established, engagement is possible.

Engaging with someone is being listened to as an equal. Whether the person with dementia is engaged in a conversation, participating in a solitary activity, or enjoying a shared interest, the benefits of being "lost in the moment" can re-create anew or re-create (from the word recreation) a feeling of a restored body and mind.

I can get totally lost in a good book and can be so unaware of the passage of time. When I eventually take a break, I realize I've missed lunch and am watching the sunset and feel so refreshed. What do you do to "get lost in time" and return with higher levels of positive emotions with an improved mood? Is it a physical activity such as working out or a passive activity such as reading, starting an art project, or perhaps golf?

How often do you tell yourself you are going to take a walk, read a book, or just find a quiet spot and relax, and none of these wonderful intentions come to fruition? Most of us, even on our best days, can talk ourselves out of doing something we might enjoy. Being able to manage our time, finding the energy and mustering up the motivation must all come together like aligning the stars.

Motivating yourself can be very difficult, especially if you are providing support for someone less motivated than you. There are times when you feel exhausted or stressed, and managing your time to implement any activity together seems almost impossible. But learning and practicing techniques for engagement can make such a difference in your and your loved one's day. Research shows that engaging people living with dementia in meaningful activities is beneficial in "increasing positive emotions, improving activities of daily living (ADL) and improving quality of life." (8)

I so often hear from family members that my loved one "just sits in the chair, watches TV, sleeps, and plays on his phone all day." They report the person may only get up to go to the bathroom after several hours of sitting. Watching television is a common interest for older people, and people over the age of 65 are watching more television than younger and middle-aged adults, but is watching TV a good option for people with dementia?

A sedentary activity, such as constant television viewing, increases the risk for obesity, cardiovascular disease, and other health concerns due to long periods of inactive physical activity for anyone, especially for those with dementia. While watching television requires little skill, is an easy diversion, and can provide periods of respite for family members, it may also be a great opportunity for engaging with your loved one. Whether you enjoy cooking, walking, or coffee together, developing a routine and scheduling times to watch favorite shows together can be an enjoyable shared activity.

People experiencing short-term memory loss may have difficulty following plots to movies or new television programs, so finding older, familiar shows that are entertaining and light-hearted tends to work. Laughing together or cheering on a favorite sports team can feel like old times.

A person with dementia does not have to stop doing the things they have enjoyed in the past. As a family member or friend who has committed to the care and support of a person living with dementia, initiating engagement is essential for keeping your family member independent longer, staying connected, and encouraging ways to increase their happiness.

Because people with neurocognitive disorders may become unmotivated due to boredom and lack the initiative to engage in an activity independently, learning how to approach the person and invite them to engage with you is important. To encourage independent engagement (activities they can do alone), you can begin an activity with the person, then tell the person that you "need to run to the bathroom, and you will be right back." Leave the person and observe if they will continue with the activity independently.

You can also observe any adaptations that can be implemented to help your loved one be successful. Return in a few minutes as you said you would and engage again. You can try this several times and for several days with the same or different activities, and by helping them feel successful, self-confidence will increase, and you may notice an increase in their focus. If the activity is familiar to the person, muscle memory can kick in, and they find themselves engaged and enjoying an old hobby. Playing familiar music they enjoy while engaging in an activity can be beneficial as well.

Recently, I was coaching a woman who was so frustrated with her husband, with early symptoms of dementia. He just sat and played on his phone. I inquired what they do together throughout the day, and she replied, "Really nothing." I asked about past hobbies her husband has enjoyed, and she replied he loved collecting stamps. She continued to tell me her son had just bought his dad new stamps, a new book, and a table magnifying glass. I asked if her husband enjoyed his stamps, and she replied, "No, but he knows where they are. I've even asked him if he wanted to look at his stamps, and he says "no."

I then asked if she sat with her husband and invited him to join her at the table to show him how to use the new magnifying glass, hoping perhaps he might show interest. He may have been intimidated by the new gadget and afraid he would not know how to use it or break the instrument. She then told me no, she had not, and explained, "I really have no interest in stamps." She missed the whole point.

Sadly, her answer was typical for family members who haven't yet gained the skills and understanding that when you commit to supporting someone with dementia, keeping them engaged in life is your responsibility. Providing essential care, such as preparing meals, personal hygiene, etc., is a given, but there is more to supporting your family member or friend than meeting basic needs. Once families and friends try a new approach to supporting their loved ones, they discover the person they are supporting is still living and not dying from dementia. As dementia progresses, the person living with dementia becomes less able to enter our world, so we must create opportunities to join theirs.

Just as the man above said no to working on his stamp collection, so often, that is the first response when a request is given to do something. Although showing respect and honoring choice is important, often, the suggestion or request is related to something they would have been willing to do in the past, such as taking a walk in the garden or looking at a stamp collection. So why do they so often respond with a "no?"

The reason is that dementia affects not just memory but language and judgment. They may not really understand what you are asking and are fearful they will fail, get lost, or embarrass themselves. We will reject suggestions if we are asked to do something we don't understand. With a little creativity, a slight shift in speech, and a bit of patience, the following strategies may be helpful in turning "no" into "yes."

Avoid yes or no questions, as it is too easy to say no. Rather than asking, "Mom, would you like to go sit outside in the garden?" instead, try, "Mom, it is so pretty outside. I would love for you to help me water the patio plants." A gentle physical prompt is also helpful. Taking their hand and walking toward the door while thanking her for her help might work.

You can also try asking a choice question. "Mom, would you like to go sit in the garden with me before or after lunch?" If the answer is after lunch, then honor that or suggest, "Let's go now, and then we can relax after lunch. Here is your sweater." Encouragement and positive facial expressions can promote more cooperation. Because of dementia, people often make poor choices regarding their health and well-being. Keeping your loved one engaged and active creates more joyful experiences to share throughout the day and provides a healthy lifestyle.

I offer phone coaching for individuals, families, and friends, and a question I get most often asked is, "What is a good activity for someone with dementia?" I get this same question during staff training in assisted living and memory care communities. I will often respond with a question: "What is a good activity for you?" They quickly start shouting out hobbies they value, events they enjoy, and places they love to go. Got it?

The activity must be meaningful to the person with dementia, just like activities need to be meaningful to you to enjoy. Often, family members (due to stigma and misunderstanding of dementia) conclude the person can "no longer do that." This makes me sad when it happens. Why should someone just determine a person living with confusion and memory loss cannot enjoy things they have always enjoyed without at least letting them try?

Engagement does not always have to be with an activity. Simply sitting at the table and having meals together will encourage better eating habits for both of you. I can't tell you how many times I hear, "I don't have time to sit down. I fixed the meal and then continued with my work (laundry, dishes). I eat when I can." Don't miss simple and natural opportunities to connect with your family members or friends.

Another strategy you can try to encourage engagement is placing visual prompts in sight around the house that may encourage the person to try an activity independently. Walking by a table with a jigsaw puzzle might prompt the person to sit down and work the puzzle. Please always keep in mind the person may engage in an activity differently than before as ability levels change. The person may sit down and just wiggle their fingers through the puzzle pieces in the box or examine the puzzle pieces and never find a fit. That is okay. Their brain is being stimulated, and they are relaxed. Our expectations must change as our loved ones' abilities change.

Displaying a variety of familiar reading materials around the home can also be helpful. A basket filled with newspapers, magazines, almanacs, or brochures will make great reading (or looking at the pictures) to keep your loved one stimulated and interested. Games are a fun and interactive way to work on a variety of cognitive skills. Tactile games like Jenga or Dominos enable those with memory challenges to use processing and motor skills, as well as socialization while playing. Remember to let them establish the rules!

Keeping a container of art supplies on hand for creative inspiration is useful for those with expressive language difficulties. Adult coloring books with colored pencils (not children's coloring books and crayons) or watercolors and art paper are easy ways to express oneself when verbal skills are not as sharp as they once were. Generally, when you sit down with the person and start an art activity, your family member will join in. Do not expect them to pick up the paintbrush and begin on their own.

Placing photo albums and framed photos out on display may create opportunities for your loved one to reminisce. This may help bring up positive emotions from enjoyable events or holidays. Be respectful if they do not recall the person's name or event. Remember, feelings, not facts! Simply look at the pictures and identify objects that may be familiar. Have fun with creating opportunities for your family members to be challenged, but always be mindful that there are never wrong answers when you are sharing time with someone with memory loss.

Creating engagement boxes for your family member is helpful in fostering meaningful engagement and creating a sense of purpose and belonging. Using a person-centered approach when developing the engagement boxes will bring success when it is specific to the individual and their capabilities. The boxes are also useful for decreasing anxiety, much like the woman's purse filled with personal comforting items. Shoeboxes are ideal, and plastic shoeboxes with lids are available at dollar discount stores. They are perfect and can be stacked for storage. You, your grandchildren, and your friends can enjoy the boxes together. Sit with the person to get them started looking through the box. Use the "I'll be right back" strategy to see if they can engage independently. Always return in a few minutes as you promised.

Theme boxes specific to your loved one might include flower arranging with artificial flowers, and a vase of live flowers are not available. Sanding blocks for the woodworker could include several 2"x4" blocks with one side covered with sandpaper, pieces of wood (different shapes) and a cloth to wipe down the sanded pieces.

An office worker might enjoy papers to fold and place in envelopes, colored paper, pencils and a pencil sharpener, a stapler, file folders, index cards, and rubber bands. A knitting box with yarn to roll into balls and needles with yarn already started (muscle memory can often kick in) for the person who has prior interest and skills.

Did your loved one enjoy coupon clipping? Include scissors, coupons and envelopes. A shoeshine box with cloth, wax (avoid the dyes), shoe strings, and a brush might be familiar. Coin sorting boxes with coins (avoid for those who may put them in their mouth), plastic coin holders, and paper rolls can also help. Gardeners may find gloves, a cap, and seeds packages as a wonderful sensory activity.

Tap into their hobbies/interests when designing the box. Use boxes that will fit comfortably on their lap if they do not want to come to a table. Engagement boxes are great fun to make and a perfect way to create joyful experiences!

# Activity

Brainstorm with family members for ideas for activity boxes and write them below. Be sure and add more ideas and create boxes specific for grandchildren to use during a visit.

# Chapter 5
## *Meeting Unmet Needs*

*"They most likely said it because they have an unmet need."* -Marshall B. Rosenberg.

What comes to mind when you read the above quote? Are you thinking of a hurtful comment your loved one said this morning while you were trying your best to help them get ready for the day? Or did an angry remark and a suddenly raised hand last evening from the person you have loved since high school bring such fear that you question whether you can continue living this way?

As you begin applying the L.O.V.E. Approach, you will become more aware of why certain "out of character" behaviors, such as swearing, impulsiveness, or mean-spirited comments from your loved one, even happen. It is very upsetting to watch your loved one turn their frustrations and confusion toward someone they love. Understanding how your loved one communicates their needs, whether through unpredictable movements, body language, or confusing comments when verbal expression is tough, you can begin to identify their need and perhaps foster a more empathetic and compassionate response to meet that need.

When a person lacks the mental, functional, or physical ability to care for themselves and can no longer meet their own needs, they must depend on someone for day-to-day support. When a family member or friend commits to providing that support for the person at home, there are basic expectations for the person. Feeling safe, both physically and emotionally, is essential for overall health and well-being. With the progression of dementia, the person's needs may increase beyond the support you can provide. Utilizing outside resources such as home health to assist with personal care or to provide opportunities for respite and exploring communities that specialize in more advanced care is wise. Keeping your family member socially engaged with friends and family members is important so your loved one will remain as active and independent as long as possible and be able to meet their own needs longer. So what are needs, and why are they important?

You may recall being introduced to Abraham Maslow's Hierarchy of Needs (1943) in junior high or high school. The visual diagram portrayed in the shape of a pyramid shows a climb from our most basic needs to the need to reach our full potential. In the simplest of terms, Maslow believed that human beings are motivated by needs, starting at the wide base of the pyramid describing our most fundamental physiological needs, such as the need for air, food, water, shelter, and clothing. The next four needs include safety, the need to love and belong, the need for self-esteem and to feel respected, and finally, the highest need to reach self-actualization and the fulfillment of your talents.

Maslow later expanded the pyramid to include cognitive, aesthetic, and transcendence needs, and although his theory was based more on philosophy rather than scientific evidence, it has great merit in understanding unmet needs in persons with dementia. It is impossible for one person (a primary support family member) to meet all the needs of someone who has lost the ability to meet even their basic needs. Thus, the involvement of friends is essential.

Addressing the symptoms of dementia requires patience. It is difficult to not overreact, correct inaccurate facts, or avoid reacting harshly to your loved one when questions are constantly repeated.

When you are doing your very best, you may feel under-appreciated from your loved one or perhaps even from other members of your family. If your needs are neglected and you are exhausted, and feel overwhelmed with the continual responsibilities, it is difficult sometimes to respond calmly and even rationally.

Language difficulties are a common symptom in people with dementia because of the changes in the brain, and comments and behaviors should not be seen as the person's fault. A hurtful comment while dressing may be an underlying feeling of a loss of independence and embarrassment because they require assistance for something as simple as putting on a shirt. An angry remark and raised hand may be an expression of frustration, being tired, or a desire to not be rushed.

So, what causes an unmet need? The Unmet Needs Model of Cohen and Mansfield states that symptoms of dementia result from an "imbalance in the interaction between lifelong habits and personality, current physical and mental states, and less than optimal environmental conditions" and "stemming from a decreased ability to communicate those needs and to provide for oneself." (9)

If your family member seems to be walking aimlessly about the house, it is likely the person has a purpose. The person may be communicating a need for engagement in an activity due to boredom or a need to do physical activity. Vocalizations from persons with dementia could be attempts to indicate pain, discomfort, or loneliness, and they are seeking human connections. Observing your loved one or friend can help you identify times of the day that trigger anxiety, restlessness, or other signs of an unmet need. How often does your family member stay by your side or walk up to you and stand next to you? Could they be seeking safety and reassurance or perhaps companionship?

Socialization is so important to reduce feelings of loneliness for both you and your family member. Socialization also helps improve self-esteem and well-being, reduces anxiety, and can reduce symptoms of depression. According to the Center for Disease Control, it is estimated that around 40% of a family member that provides the most support to a person living with dementia has two or more chronic illnesses, and around 35% of persons over the age of 65 have a disability. Studies continue to indicate that family members and friends of a person living with dementia benefit from training specific to address their own health and psychosocial well-being.

Support strategies to promote feelings of success and well-being for your family member can be as simple as giving one directive or request at a time if the person has difficulty doing more than one task at a time. For example, rather than asking the person to put on their socks and shoes, start by suggesting they put on a sock. Once that has been accomplished, then prompt the person to put on a shoe. If the person has difficulty solving problems or making decisions, give two solutions or solve the problem together and practice patience so a person has time to complete a physical or cognitive task. "Learned helplessness" results when someone is "unable to exercise reasonable mastery in one situation incorrectly assumes that he or she is then unable to exercise reasonable control in other situations," and they will stop trying. (10)

Learning to listen, observe, validate, and engage in meaningful connections will help identify and address the unmet needs of your loved one. But what about you? Are your needs being met? How do you express your unmet needs, and what happens when your needs are not being met? If two words were changed in the quote at the beginning of the chapter and it read like this, "I most likely said it because I have an unmet need," would that sound familiar?

Do your comments or actions, as a response to your loved ones' comments or actions, result in a hurtful statement and create a conflict? Do you catch yourself wishing you could have a do-over when perhaps you reacted too harshly because you are tired or feeling resentment toward your loved one? Do you feel remorse when you see the hurt or shame on your loved one's face when you unintentionally correct or embarrass him or her and realize you just need a good cry?

Identifying your needs and achieving a balance in how to meet those needs is a big step in practicing self-care. Learning to ask for help from family and friends is a sign of strength and courage, not defeat. When you become more aware of your own unmet needs and are able to attach words to a feeling, such as anger, sadness, loneliness, resentment, or simply being overwhelmed, you can begin to make sense of your emotions and meet your own unmet needs more easily.

A very simple technique I started practicing in the early 1980s to stay in check with my emotions while working as a therapist in addiction and mental health is to H.A.L.T. By pausing and quickly assessing and asking if I am Hungry, Angry, Lonely, or Tired can help identify a change in my mood. If you are familiar with a 12-step program, you will recognize this acronym that was developed to help addicts in recovery, identify triggers, and prevent a relapse. Taking a moment to take a deep breath and H.A.L.T. may help avoid a conflict the next time you begin to see a shift in your mood. Questioning if you are thirsty should be included in the "hungry" assessment because becoming dehydrated can cause mood swings, headaches, urinary tract infections, and confusion.

This, of course, is a quick and simple way to assess your family members as well when they experience a change in mood. People with dementia may be unable to let you know they need water, and dehydration can cause increased confusion. Signs can be constipation, dizziness, dark urine, or a dry mouth. Often, people living with dementia will forget to drink water. Even offering a glass of water to the person does not always mean they will drink it. Making sure your loved one receives the best care possible starts with meeting basic needs.

Understanding your personality and your thoughts, emotions, beliefs, reactions, and your relationship with others will help identify your strengths and improve your ability to manage your emotions and have more control over your life. Developing self-awareness can make you a better communicator, manage and regulate your emotions, and your confidence in decision-making skills.

Learning techniques for developing self-awareness was an essential skill introduced early in my career. I loved working in the mental health and substance abuse field, and the skills I learned have been invaluable, influencing my personal and professional life. Being trained in crisis intervention techniques, group facilitation, identifying unmet needs, and problem-solving creatively has served me well in every job, with every person, and with every family I have been honored to serve.

Because alcoholism (addiction) affects all family members, not just the addict, family members tend to fall into survival roles, and like the addict, family members need treatment as well to heal and process the chaos and unpredictability of living in a dysfunctional home. I had the pleasure of hearing the renowned author Claudia Black Ph.D., speak in the early 1980's and was introduced to the "three unspoken rules" in a dysfunctional family such as a family living with addiction. In her book, *It Will Never Happen to Me*, she explains that dysfunctional families follow three unspoken rules: Don't talk, don't trust, and don't feel.

While working in addiction, these three simple rules were so evident in the family systems and the effects of childhood trauma from growing up in a dysfunctional home. "Don't talk" refers to the fear of letting others know the family secrets, outsiders, or even to each other. This included the denial and attempt to look "normal." The "don't trust" rule results from the inconsistency and unpredictable stress, neglect, and lack of understanding that needs are not always being met. And the third unwritten rule, "don't feel," is confusing because feelings are not validated. Thus, family members learn to repress feelings.

From my experiences and observations throughout my career, I have seen these three simple rules informally appear in dysfunctional work settings, social groups, and families living with dementia or Alzheimer's disease. Please note: This is only my observation, but I do see so many families supporting someone with cognitive decline who "don't talk" about the diagnosis to friends and even other family members. Perhaps it is due to the stigma that dementia brings, but these families also "don't trust" others, even healthcare professionals. Hesitations to truthfully express what is going on in the home encompasses the "don't feel" rule. Feelings may be minimized or criticized by others, and we often neglect to validate our loved one's feelings, much less our own.

Providing support at home can impact everyday life, and how dementia affects the family and individual family members varies. Allowing you, your family and friends, and your loved one living with dementia to talk about the life changes a dementia diagnosis brings, to trust others to share in your life and encourage the expression of feelings, communication improves, resilience increases, and the connections with yourself and others can be more honest and genuine.

People living with dementia need support, not just the basic needs, but also the need to feel they belong and feel safe and respected, such as helping the person find purpose in each day. The idea of learning new skills and finding new "tools" must feel overwhelming at times. According to a cross-sectional survey of persons with dementia, the primary support person, and health care professionals, the most frequent needs "were in the areas of daytime activities, company, and psychological stress." (11)

If there are respite services or day programs available in your area, these resources can help meet the social needs of your family member and allow time for you to take a break. Recently, a gentleman living with dementia was attending a respite program I was facilitating. When his wife arrived to pick him up, I was eager to tell her how talkative and social he was all morning. When I shared his day with her, she only replied with a question: "But did he eat his lunch?" Ensuring his basic needs are met seemed to be her only consideration. Perhaps that was all she could do.

When you use the tools of the L.O.V.E. Approach, you will begin to recognize a positive difference in the relationship with your loved one or friend. When we have limited tools, we tend to rely on the same ineffective coping skills used in the past. By practicing the L.O.V.E. Approach consistently, you begin to experience a new way of thinking and responding to reoccurring challenges more effectively. You and your loved one or friend can move beyond the base of Maslow's pyramid and focus on more advanced needs such as emotional connections, engaging in meaningful activities, and within the ability levels of your loved one, help him or her find their purpose in life.

*"If the only tool you have is a hammer, you tend to see every problem as a nail."*
-Abraham Maslow

## Activity 1

Take a few moments and think about needs that you have that are not being met. The need to socialize, get some sleep, or the need for alone time? Then, brainstorm how your unmet needs can be addressed.

## Activity 2

What are some examples where you listened, observed, validated or engaged with your loved one?

## Chapter 6
## Who am I? Who are you?

*"You are not my caregiver; you are my wife."* -husband with Alzheimer's disease.

Having a strong sense of identity by knowing who we are and what we believe provides direction in our lives, creates self-awareness, gives us a perspective of our values, and helps us stay grounded. Understanding ourselves also helps us make sense of our world and where we belong. Our identities are unique and complex because we form our self-identity from our life experiences, family upbringing, culture, work experience, relationships, personality, and memories. Self-identity influences our aspirations and the gifts, talents, and superpowers we share with others.

Besides our identity, we embrace roles throughout our lives that are constantly changing. Family roles can change during significant events. Taking on the role of a mother or father after the birth of a child, and years later, a new role may unfold to include being a grandparent. Other than the family roles we acquire, we have our personal roles that encompass our self-growth and well-being, our professional and social roles, and the role we serve in our community.

Changing roles in our family can be joyful but also sad and difficult. For instance, families will often become closer and learn the importance of supporting each other when a significant loss or death occurs. When a grandparent, parent, or sibling dies, it can affect how we see ourselves. Do we take on the responsibility a sibling may have had that influenced the dynamics of the family? Or how do we understand the loss of a parent and the role we have played as a daughter or son? As roles change in our families, we find that life goes on, even though things are not the same.

Seeing ourselves as a whole person, and not just one facet of our life, helps create a positive sense of self. Our values and beliefs influence how we see ourselves and understand where we belong and how our relationships shape us. The contributions we make to others, our communities, and our world are part of ourselves and tie into our purpose in life. We also identify with what others think of us and what we call ourselves. We may not want that identity and can fall into the trap of how society sees us. Our identity is who we really are, not the role we play.

The Caregiver Identity Theory (Montgomery and Kosloski 2009) suggests that our role as a caregiver evolves from an existing role as a family member or friend and the transition of the role during the progression of cognitive decline. The theory suggests that transitions are in phases, and the first phase begins with a family member or friend gradually taking on tasks that the family member living with memory loss usually does for the family. It is such a subtle change and is before a diagnosis or even suspicion that something is changing in the person, and the changes are dismissed due to aging.

The phases continue in increments as more assistance is given, and eventually, the role will evolve beyond the typical role and relationship you have with the person. As the responsibilities increase, by the third and fourth phases, significant help is required that goes farther than the boundaries of the relationship, such as providing personal care. During these phases, the support and constant required care change the relationship of the person providing care and may begin to identify as a "caregiver."

The significance of the changing roles may determine when the person may or may not seek help or when healthcare professionals need to intervene. Research continues to explore why families don't reach out for help in the early stages of a dementia diagnosis. Some thoughts are the stigma, lack of education, and fear of a diagnosis. Lacking the awareness of symptoms and resistance from the person to seek help also contributes to a delay in a diagnosis. When healthcare providers professionals can offer the needed services at the required time during the progression of the cognitive decline, more families and friends may reach out and benefit from services earlier.

New names have been created for those who did not want to be seen as "caregivers," such as "care partner," "care provider," or "carers." All of the terms explain what this person does for their loved one, but it is not who they are. Another term that is often used is "caretaker." The term originated in England, and a "caretaker" did indeed take care of the sick. But the newer term "caregiver" evolved in the US, and now "caretakers" are generally people who "take care" of "buildings, animals, or graves." Who knew?

Identifying as a "caregiver" can create an imbalance of power, and the person with dementia can lose autonomy and personhood, feel powerless, become depressed, and give up. Spouses, sons, and daughters often report that losing their identity is one of the hardest consequences to overcome during the time they care for someone. Maintaining your identity and relationship with your loved one is important. When you only identify as a caregiver, you limit yourself to the world of caregiving. Understanding that you are caregiving but continuing to see yourself as who you are and not see yourself by what you do is key to maintaining your identity.

When the dynamics of a relationship change, and one person in the relationship becomes dominant, it is called power dynamics, describing the power between two or more people. This person of power makes decisions for another person that affect the other person's life and can determine the amount and quality of care given when providing support. The person living with dementia is at risk of losing his/her own identity when this occurs. It is important to understand that anytime someone is reliant on care from another person, there will be a power dynamic in that relationship. When you see yourself in family roles, respect each other, and refrain from using power to gain cooperation, you will create a less confrontative and controlling environment.

Another consequence of identifying totally as a caregiver may not be apparent until after the caregiving is complete and you find yourself in an identity crisis. Giving up who you are and putting yourself on hold affects you emotionally and physically and can lead to serious negative health outcomes.

Continuing with the relationship roles you have with the individual with dementia shows respect and honors their dignity. By using a strengths-based approach by building on their strengths, modifying tasks, and focusing on what the person can do rather than can't do, persons with dementia can maintain independence longer, and the person continues to feel a sense of purpose in life. Breaking the stigma of "suffering from dementia" and starting seeing your family member or friend as "living with dementia," you can continue to maintain relationships as a spouse, daughter, son, grandchild, or friend.

Working in hospital and clinical settings as a therapist, I wasn't familiar with the term "caregiver" until 1997, when I left clinical settings and began working in the community with children and young adults with physical and developmental disabilities and their families. I was more familiar with nurses, therapists, doctors, and CNAs.

I learned quickly that these families who had a child with a disability were referred to as "caregivers" in the school system, and families disliked that term profusely. They saw themselves as moms and dads raising their children with love and hope like other parents; their children just happened to have a disability. One of the first moms I met explained to me that the "special education" department at the child's school referred to her as her child's "primary caregiver" for the purpose of the IEP (Individualized Education Plan). She was so upset and asked the school staff to change the terminology, but the school refused.

I met many wonderful families during this time and keep up with some moms on social media and enjoy watching their children grow into productive adults. The mother of a ten-year-old son with Down syndrome told me when the nurse put her son in her arms, the doctor was there to tell her of the child's "condition." There was little information or even hope for a child with a disability to live a meaningful life at that time, and she was totally overwhelmed. Her plans to have a neurotypical child who could grow up and be a football star, have a job he loved, and marry and have a family of his own were suddenly changed; however, today, her son is an accomplished athlete and happy and healthy today, with a girlfriend.

But these parents, just as you are doing, acquired the skills to address the specific needs of their child and give their child a life of quality. They grieved the loss of the future they planned with the child, just as you grieve for the loss of the future you had planned with your loved one or friend. These moms and dads and brothers and sisters have challenges along the way to support the child with a disability and can become empowered and live a meaningful and purposeful life together. These parents taught me a very valuable lesson that was reinforced years later when my own mother became chronically ill.

Maintaining your identity and the relationship with your loved one or friend is important for both you and the person living with dementia. It is also very important that you don't experience a "loss of self." if you become immersed in a "caregiver" role. Younger adults, females, and spouses are at a higher risk for this to occur. (12)

The AARP Public Policy Institute's Caregiving in the US 2020 report found that 53% of caregivers felt they had no choice when becoming a caregiver, and 51% said that a caregiver role gave them meaning in their lives with a sense of purpose. The report did note that even with the group of caregivers who felt a sense of purpose, the findings stated they still felt feelings of loneliness and financial, physical, and emotional strain.

## Spousal Relationships

When my parents married on June 16, 1952, they pledged to "have and to hold from this day forward, for better, for worse, for richer, for poorer, in sickness and in health, to love and to cherish, until parted by death." That was their solemn vow.

I witnessed that vow for 38 years, during the good times and some tough times, until my mother's death in 1994. By definition, my parents were "perfectly suited to each other" in temperament and unconditional love, and I believe, by definition, they were "soulmates." However, with her sheepish little grin, my mother always attributed the longevity of their relationship to "no one else would have your father."

My parents were fortunate to be married for 42 years and, overall, were happy together. As in all families, we had our struggles and some very difficult times, but somehow, my parents always came together when parenting three daughters and were able to raise three self-reliant women. Studies show married people live longer and are healthier than people who are single, and it is suggested the companionship, stability, and predictability of a relationship are significant factors.

My parents built my childhood home in 1954, and like most families in that era, we had a car, a cat, and a dog. And while some houses were adorned with a white picket fence, our chain link fence in the backyard was much more suitable for our Saint Bernard, whom my dad brought home as a puppy. Mom had asked my dad to find a "small indoor dog," and although my two sisters and I were not involved in the selection of our family pet, we were very pleased with Dad's choice.

My easygoing, dry-witted mother, of course, was a bit taken back but welcomed the giant puppy and declared he was a SNAFU, a military term my dad would use: "Situation Normal, All Fouled Up." So Snafu became part of the family for much of my childhood, and because of my dad's "little snafu" when I was 10 years old, my love for canine companions continues, and thus, I have always shared my home with a dog(s). Pets can be very therapeutic, so if you don't have a dog or cat, connect with a neighbor or friend to bring theirs for a visit weekly with your family member..

I was raised in a playful, funny, and loud family. I was always curious and creative and loved to play. I have always been a tinkerer and thrived when discovering ways to express my creativity and find innovative ways to do things a bit differently. This has served me well. It is obvious to me now why creativity has been my superpower throughout my life. I had many side hustles growing up: teaching guitar lessons, mowing yards, making jewelry, and briefly selling cinnamon toothpick sticks on the black market to junior high school peers.

In the 1980's, my mother had a life-threatening event and was intubated and placed on life support. It was heartbreaking that she was never able to wean off the ventilator, and when she became strong enough to leave the hospital, the discharge planning team arranged for a bed in a skilled nursing facility. She was alert and very cognizant and expressed she wanted to return home.

When we told the doctor our plan to take her back home, they objected and explained that it was impossible because of her serious medical needs. That answer did not work for us. We fought tooth and nail, and the physicians and administrators finally agreed, but with strict guidelines for her safety and ours. Dad purchased the gas generator they required in case my parents home lost power, and we all took a CPR class for someone on a ventilator and learned how to suction her tracheostomy. We were the first family from that hospital to bring someone home on a ventilator.

My point? None of us identified as a caregiver. We simply learned the skills to keep my mother safe. We knew nothing about being caregivers, but we did know how to be sisters, daughters, a husband, and a father. I don't think my dad even knew the word caregiver. He was her husband and our dad. He brought her flowers, teased how much he loved his first wife (he was only married to my mother), cooked, cleaned, and did the laundry while continuing to live the vows he declared four decades prior. They would watch movies together and hold hands like nothing had changed.

Professional caregivers came throughout the week for personal care and to monitor her vitals. This was a big adjustment for my parents because they were a private couple. It was especially difficult on my mom because my dad was always around, and she never really had any alone time.

When you are supporting someone with cognitive decline, relationships can change. One woman I recently met told me the Alzheimer's diagnosis for her husband has been a blessing. She reports he is more loving and affectionate, and they are closer than they ever have been. You never know how dementia is going to affect the person or your relationship.

When recognizing changes in someone's behavior, such as confusion about time or place or the person is having difficulty with common everyday tasks, early memory loss may be the reason. When a spouse notices these changes in his/her loved one, they may make excuses and deny that something is changing.

He/she will begin taking on more responsibility for the person's tasks, such as helping pick out clothes or answering for the person to avoid the chance that the person may not be able to respond approximately. He/she will then attempt to convince other family members that "mom is just getting old" because of fear it could be dementia. This avoidance technique can last for years, and a diagnosis may eventually come, but help is often "too little too late."

The consequences of untreated dementia over a long period of time can result in total social isolation, faster decline in abilities, and injuries, and the person can be at risk of hurting themselves or others. Denial is a coping mechanism used to protect ourselves, and it will often give us a period to adjust to the new circumstances and allow us time to process this new reality. But hopefully, the person in denial will eventually become more aware of the situation and gain the strength to seek help.

But often, even when behaviors associated with memory loss are so apparent to others, the spouse won't come to terms with the "elephant in the room," and the person with dementia misses out on early treatment that could affect their long-term health. A spouse with dementia may become physical in an attempt to communicate a need or become so withdrawn that connecting and engaging may be impossible. The L.O.V.E. Approach cannot be all things to all people, but if you have the basic understanding to listen, observe, validate, and engage, you can learn to problem solve and perhaps be better prepared for the changes that occur.

Spouses of someone living with dementia are often isolated from friends and feel a sense of loss, even when the spouse is still living. Spousal caregivers experiencing caregiver strain have also been shown to have mortality risks that are 63 percent higher than non-caregivers. But which spouse provides the best care? Studies suggest it is not necessarily based on gender but related more to the dynamics of the relationship. The more dominant spouse will often fail to address the concerns and emotions of the non-dominant spouse because they often lack empathy and compassion and maintain control of the providing care throughout the illness.

The non-dominant spouse, on the other hand, is often caring and empathetic and responds to the needs and demands of the person, but often out of fear or intimidation of the dominant spouse. When a person with dementia is controlling and demanding, constant power struggles are a daily challenge. It is imperative to avoid power struggles by leaving the room and taking a break or getting additional support.

Asserting power and control over a spouse (or anyone) involves manipulation, blaming, shaming, and yelling and, many times, is a result of the person's own insecurities. Living in an environment where you are constantly belittled, threatened, controlled, and insulted creates an emotionally abusive relationship and can be a serious concern for the safety and well-being of the person being emotionally attacked with hurtful words or threats.

During these times, the person giving the care can naturally become angry, but being able to manage and self-regulate emotions is essential. People with dementia are sensitive to your feelings and mood and react to your anxiety. You want to avoid any physical altercation, no matter what. But if you are experiencing physical or continued emotional abuse, this is very serious, regardless if the person's behavior is beyond their control due to dementia, and you need to seek help. Women can, of course, be emotionally abusive to men, but women experience a higher rate of this type of abuse.

Please find the help you need if you are in a situation of any kind of abuse because the abuse can cause short and long-term and detrimental health consequences, both physical and emotional. I have worked with women who experienced emotional (and physical) abuse during the caregiving years, and some women admitted they experienced psychological abuse throughout the marriage, and dementia just made it worse.

There has to be a partnership between spouses. Keeping your loved one's personhood intact is fundamental for person-centered care. "Persons with dementia cannot be assumed to be incapable of making decisions on the basis of their diagnosis alone as they may have retained abilities." ( 13 )

## Adult Children and Relationships

Adult children of aging parents may become involved in the care of one or both parents if changes in their health and safety become a concern. Oftentimes, the parents live away from their children, and an adult child may decide to move closer to the parent(s), live with the parent(s), invite the parent(s) to move closer to them, or even live with their family. The geographical proximity or gender of an adult child can influence which child voluntarily or involuntarily takes on the role of supporting the parent(s).

Circumstances will differ for each family, and sacrifices are made by all. Parents may willingly move closer to the adult child who has committed to the care, or the adult child may uproot the parents unwillingly from their home, friends, and community for the parent(s) well-being or sometimes merely for the adult child's convenience. It may be the best option in the long run, and hopefully, proper care and support will be given. However, I have worked with many older couples who "had to move" because of their son or daughter's demands and the relationships suffered.

Change is hard on older individuals. Having your parents move to an unfamiliar place is very frightening. Nevertheless, either scenario is a life-changing event for all involved, so understanding the resistance from your parent is based on fear, not the goal of being "obstinate." Their fear of losing their independence and the overwhelming feeling of packing up and leaving a home and community they love is a profound emotional shift in their future. Spending money and paying their own way is often a worry for older adults. Being fearful of outspending their assets is a senior's biggest fear, regardless of how much money they have.

When a parent of an adult child is experiencing cognitive declines, such as changes in memory, judgment, language, and thinking skills, decision-making, and even financial obligations may fall on the child. Concerns about falls, money management, wandering, and overall safety can be overwhelming and are common, especially if the adult child lives out of town. It is also not uncommon to find a parent has more debt than they have disclosed.

At times, the adult child will take on the mindset that the parent/child roles have been reversed and they are now "parenting" their mother or father. This is a dangerous attitude because it implies their parent has reverted to childhood, and they begin treating the person like a child. Parents discipline and make most decisions for their children because that's their job. But when an adult child falls into this belief, neglect and abuse can happen.

A couple had been attending one of my groups for over three years. They were both in their eighties, and the wife had been providing sole support for her husband, who had Alzheimer's disease, for several years. Unfortunately, she took a fall and died suddenly. Her death resulted in an unexpected move for a daughter into her father's home. The daughter brought in her own furniture and immediately began rearranging the house, confusing her father as he was trying to process the sudden disappearance of his wife. Apparently, this daughter had spent little time with her parents and lacked even basic knowledge of dementia. At her mother's funeral, she told me, almost giddily, how much she was enjoying "yelling at my father" as a means of payback for times he raised his voice at her when she was going up. I offered her my condolences and assistance if she needed any. I reached out once to her but did not hear back. Her father died a few weeks later, perhaps from a broken heart.

It is estimated that roughly 30% of older spouses caring for someone with dementia will die before the person they are caring for. A UC Berkley study published in the Proceedings of the National Academy of Sciences journal showed that a person being cared for by someone with high anxiety, depression, or other mental health concerns will die sooner than those who are cared for by someone with good mental health.

Adult children experience feelings of frustration, powerlessness, abandonment, and sorrow when they attempt to engage with their parents the way they always have failed. Adult children long for the past relationship and the comfort and safety a parent may have provided. On the other hand, if there was a contentious relationship prior to the diagnosis, resentment and anger may become more apparent by both the parent and adult child.

It is possible that by taking on the responsibility of supporting a parent in an estranged relationship with a child, healing can occur. However, if this is not possible, the vulnerable parent is at risk of not receiving the proper care they require. If an adult child (or anyone) takes on the care of a parent because of guilt, obligation, financial gain, or other nefarious reasons, the quality of care can be compromised.

When adult children recognize the parent's needs require more support and really do want the best for them, insisting they move closer can bring great resistance. The child may view their parent's unwillingness to cooperate as being stubborn and selfish rather than recognizing the parent is just trying to stand up for their rights. Taking a slower approach to the idea of moving closer to "the grandkids" or family, parents may be less defensive. Presenting the idea, then stepping back so they can process the information and bring it up again later may make for a smoother transition and avert relationships from becoming fractured.

Adult children need to be included in the diagnostic portion phase and gain as much understanding of the parent's diagnosis as possible. Having someone join the spouse to the doctor's visit is also important in order to have correct information regarding the prognosis, medications, and perhaps supporting the other parent. Sometimes, the adult child and the parent without dementia do not see eye to eye on the care or treatment the parent with dementia is receiving. When you need to address the concern of the parent with dementia and the other parent is just not ready, avoid demanding that the parent come to terms with the memory loss. Ask to have a conversation, even when the topic is uncomfortable. You may find that he/she is relieved to talk about it.

Try to understand the fears that prevent a spouse from coming to terms with memory loss. Are they fearful they would be separated from each other? Perhaps fearful of the long-term consequences of dementia? Learn the symptoms of cognitive impairment and share them with your parent. Keeping a journal of the behavioral changes may help others recognize a change in cognitive abilities. Always remember the importance of self-care and attend a family support group for dementia. If none of these suggestions work, don't hesitate too long before asking for professional help.

For adult children with a parent diagnosed with a type of dementia, the child is not only fearful of the outcome for the parent but knows the reality they have the possibility of understanding dementia can run in families. The Centers for Disease Control reports that family history can increase your risk for developing Alzheimer's disease, but only by 10% to 30%. Research indicates that approximately one-third of dementia diagnoses could be attributed to modifiable risk factors such as diabetes, mild hypertension, obesity, smoking, depression, social isolation, and lack of stimulation.

When an adult child makes a commitment to provide home care for a parent living with dementia, enormous responsibilities come with great consequences if proper care is not provided. A daughter who always had a strained relationship with her mother moved in with her to provide care when she could not care for herself because of her cognitive decline. The daughter shared with me she felt her mother "wasn't working hard enough" during her PT appointments for balance and strength to reduce fall risk, so she quit taking her mother to the appointments.

She continued telling me her mom was not motivated to do her home exercises. It was obvious this adult child did not understand dementia, and due to her mother's memory loss, she no longer had the capacity not only to remember to do the home exercises, but it is doubtful she could remember how to do them properly. Her daughter then stated almost defiantly, "I don't have time to help her with that anyway." Sadly, her mother was using a walker within a month and fell a month later, breaking her hip.

Everyone has the right to set boundaries for their own health and well-being, and adult children face difficult choices. You have the choice in the amount of involvement or the choice of no involvement in the care of your parent(s), but if you commit to being the sole support for your parent, you are responsible for respecting their rights and for the person to make their own decisions as long as they are capable. If you have power of attorney, it does not mean you have power over the person but rather the power to make the best decisions for the person who entrusted you to do so. Disregarding a prescribed treatment from a physician because you thought the person wasn't benefiting is passive neglect. In this situation, speaking to the physicians to see if other alternative approaches could help her mother's fall risk would be appropriate.

It can be easy and unintentional to fall into a pattern of passive neglect when supporting someone who is dependent on you by disregarding their ability to make decisions such as food preferences or denying a need for socialization and isolating the person in the home. The person can become a victim of financial exploitation, denied foods of preference or the right to receive proper healthcare. Passive neglect results when the support person fails to understand the person's needs and fails to meet those needs. Honoring the person's values, even if different from yours, may be difficult, but not being able to honor their values results in resentment and feelings of helplessness.

Providing support at home can be trying for adult children who have their own families to consider and are perhaps still working. I encourage you to reach out for help when you find you are unable to reasonably meet the needs of a parent who is depending on you to provide a meaningful life.

Parents instill values and expectations in their children. My mom was an avid reader, and my dad was a politician and an advocate for voting rights. Those values are very important to me now. When I move to a new city, I first obtain a library card (thank you, Mom), and secondly, I register to vote ( thank you, Dad). I got a little chuckle with a recent move. The voting precinct was in my library.

As mentioned earlier, my father was a Marine who served his country proudly. He sustained an injury to a foot during his service and walked with a significant limp, but he never felt sorry for himself, even though I know he lived with chronic pain. Besides teaching his girls about the responsibility to vote, he modeled the importance of respecting those who served to defend our democracy. We were taught always to place our hand over our hearts when we pledged alliance to our country and to stand up when the Marine Corps hymn was played, regardless of where we happened to be.

Several years ago, I was sitting on a hillside along with hundreds of others enjoying a July 4th celebration concert. We all sat and listened to the peppy music and lyrics of the United States Armed Forces Medley. I listened attentively as the orchestra played and the chorus sang, honoring the Army, Navy, Coast Guard, and Air Force. I prepared myself to stand as I always had, waiting for those commanding five words describing the historical site of the Battle of Chapultepec, "From the Halls of Montezuma." When I stood, the gentleman seated on the ground next to me inquired if I was a Marine, and I told him I stand for my father. He stood beside me, and in a matter of seconds, the row of people began to rise. I tell this because it is a wonderful and meaningful lesson in the power of one.

My mom died of pneumonia after living 18 months on life support. My dad became very depressed as he had lost his soulmate, leisure partner, and best friend. He was lost. However, Dad's mother was still living and gave him purpose. In her mid-90s, my grandmother had a stroke that left her unable to walk. My aunt, my dad's sister, moved in with my grandmother and became the "primary caregiver." My aunt was demanding, impatient, and controlling and had little patience with my grandmother, and my grandmother had little power in decision-making.

On the other hand, my dad always had a loving relationship with his mother and continued to be kind and patient. He maintained that relationship and continued being her son. He would visit regularly, giving my aunt respite opportunities. I never heard a harsh word from my dad toward his mother. He would take his mother's flowers like he did my mom and cook and deliver her favorite meals.

My dad took my grandmother fishing on her 95th birthday and she always looked forward to dad's visit. My aunt was likely jealous of the relationship my dad had with his mom, and my aunt's controlling nature could not stand for my grandmother, who was a lifelong smoker, to smoke. My aunt's refusal for my grandmother to have access to cigarettes is a great example of the imbalance of power and the control a "caregiver" can have over a person. Smoking is certainly not part of a healthy lifestyle, but my grandmother still had the right to smoke. Just because my aunt disapproved of my grandmother's lifestyle choice, she denied my grandmother's right with passive neglect.

One day, my father shared with me the routine when visiting his mother. He would wheel my grandmother outside to see her garden, where he and his mom would share a cigarette. Because her face was drawn on one side due to the stroke, she would hold the cigarette between her lips and her gnarled, arthritic fingers and always look at my dad as she took the draw. As she blew out the smoke, she would remark like clockwork, "Aww, that's good," giving my dad a head shake and a crooked little smile. She died at the ripe old age of ninety-nine, and I know how grateful she and my dad were to be able to maintain their loving relationship until the end.

Another example of passive neglect was when I was coaching a son who cared for his mother with dementia. The son valued his health and ate a very strict, healthy diet, serving his mom the same meals. He told me she was not eating and had lost weight. He did say she ate well one night a week when he "allowed" her to eat a fast-food hamburger. I know how much this woman loves her hamburgers, and she told me she would be happier if she could have a hamburger three or four times a week. I had her share this with her son, but he would not budge. If having several hamburger meals during the week could improve this woman's quality of life, I say bring on the burgers. She is ninety-four years old, for goodness sake.

## Grandparents

Grandparents have always played an important role in families, but due to changes in the past forty-five years, the responsibility of grandparents is increasing. Grandparents and older adults are an invaluable asset and provide more financial support for their families than ever before. Millions of older Americans have returned to the workforce due to fixed incomes and rising costs.

According to a recent Pew Research Center survey, Americans in their forties are "sandwiched" between their children and one or more aging parents. This "sandwich generation," with multigenerational family members living together, is becoming more common. Raising children while also supporting a parent with dementia is not out of the ordinary.

Another home situation that is growing is grandparents raising grandchildren. More than 13 million grandchildren are being raised by grandparents or other older adults because the parent (adult child of the grandparent) is living with an addiction or a mental illness and does not have the skills to parent a child. Many of these adult children are in prison, and the care is left to the grandparents, who may be struggling with their own health issues. We think of our grandparents as being at the highest risk of having dementia. However, I coached a ninety-one-year-old grandmother whose seventy-year-old daughter has dementia. The daughter lives in a community with 24-hour care, but her mother is devoted and visits her daughter as often as she can.

## Grandchildren

Young children are resilient. They are also curious, honest, and observant and often, family members think that a grandchild won't notice dementia in a grandparent. Trying to cover up for Grandpa's change in behavior by responding, "Grandpa is just joking around," or blaming it on old age, experts say that without direct answers, children reach their own conclusions, which can be frightening to them. When a child is seeing one thing and being told another, the results can often cause anxiety in the child.

Understanding dementia or Alzheimer's disease as a child or adolescent can be difficult, but having open communication will help the child feel a sense of security and overall well-being. Explaining to the child that Grandpa has an illness in his brain and cannot remember things, which makes it hard for him to do some things he used to do, may help the child understand.

Assure the child he/she cannot "catch" the illness and that they can still play with his/her grandparent. Explain what is happening when the child sees something that Grandpa does or says. Grandpa may have confused words when asking for something. Be truthful with age-appropriate answers and help the child find activities to continue staying connected with Grandpa. Explaining to a 14-year-old grandchild why Grandpa needs someone to help him bathe or helping a 5-year-old grandchild understand why Grandpa cannot make his famous cookies anymore can be explained in terms that they can understand.

In an earlier chapter, I encouraged you to discover your "superpower," or the inner strength that gets you through difficult times. I do an exercise in my practice to encourage self-awareness and to empower people to realize their powers within. One activity I use is for the participants to use aluminum foil and actually create their own Superhero. The aluminum foil sculpture is then taped to an index card, and the person names their power on the card. It is a fun and meaningful exercise, and the process ends with a little foil trophy. I have done this with college students, parents, people with dementia, and children and adolescents.

I was working with a children's pediatric cancer program and did this activity with the siblings of a child who had cancer. The siblings ranged from 9-12 in age, and during the class, they worked hard exploring their superpowers and creating the little aluminum foil statue. The children proudly shared their powers and showed the group the Superhero sculpture they had created. One young 11-year-old girl did the exercise, and when she shared her Superhero with the group, she held up the card where the aluminum sculpture should be standing, and her card was empty. She made such intentionally prolonged eye contact with me, as if she knew I could be trusted to help her and stated, "My superpower is that I am invisible."

When asked to talk more about that, she replied if she was invisible, she could sneak up on her parents and find out how sick her little brother really was. She could find out the truth about what was happening to her younger sibling she loved, and she was very aware her parents had been lying to her, telling her he was "just sick." She had overheard the whispers of her parents trying to protect her, but she knew her little brother was dying.

When I shared this with the director of the program and suggested her parents thought they were keeping his cancer a secret, the director confirmed my observation. She had been encouraging the parents to share this with their daughter, but they felt she didn't need to know. With the urging of the director, the girl's parents came clean, and her superpower was no longer needed. The risk of trusting is hard, and building trust takes time, but I am glad she felt safe with me that evening.

Children know more than you think they know, and if you don't validate what they are seeing and hearing and explain the reason in terms they can understand, they will come to their own conclusions and think that it may be their fault Grandpa is acting funny.

Be creative and develop a list of activities for them to do together so you are not caught off guard and can offer a fun experience at a moment's notice to minimize anxiety for both. Activities for them to do together can include singing, reading to each other, watching animal videos, playing musical instruments together, or watching the birds on the feeders while enjoying a snack.

I'll introduce you to my "triple play" technique I use to get two people engaged in an activity together. The person, perhaps you, sits down with the grandchild and grandpa and starts an activity, prompting how the child could engage with the grandparent. Once the two of them are engaged and connected, you pull out. Check back occasionally to validate and encourage engagement. Voila! The magic of the triple play!

You can visit your library and find books that explain dementia to children. There are many appropriate books for younger children and chapter books for adolescents. Most importantly, reinforce that no matter how confused Grandpa is and may not remember your name sometimes, "He loves you very much." Helping children understand dementia can teach the child patience and empathy and minimize any fears the child may have.

But what about older grandchildren? Often, as grandchildren get older, they may lose interest in the relationship with a grandparent, and the childhood closeness they share may wane. In a social group I facilitate for people with dementia and a family member, one ninety-two-year-old gentleman brings his college-age grandson when he visits on spring break, and they really enjoy the group and each other.

## Neighbors

During a lunch date with a good friend, she shared another friend's concerns about a neighbor who was experiencing memory loss and confusion, forgetting two lunch dates. The friend's neighbor lives alone, and her only daughter lives out of state. My friend wanted some guidance on how to approach the situation. I met my friend seven years ago during a time when she was caring for her mother, who was living with Alzheimer's disease in her home. Her mom has since passed away. She was a delightful lady and was always friendly when I visited.

My friend has a brother who was living out of town during his mother's illness, and he never visited his mother after the diagnosis. He did call his mother regularly, so I became a source of support for my friend and a safe place to vent her frustrations from receiving little support from her only sibling. I asked my friend to remind me how her mother's diagnosis came about. She told me her mother was living alone out of state, and they regularly spoke on the phone. It was generally small talk, and according to her mom, "everything was fine." People with dementia can use "pat phrases" in response to questions they may not have the answer for or do not want to answer and can become chameleons, changing their behaviors to please others.

Although my friend spoke to her mom almost daily, she had not visited in a couple of years and had not picked up on anything that might be concerning until her mother called and told her that her electricity had been turned off. My friend called the utility department and was told the bill had not been paid for three months, and they had no choice but to turn off the power. Her mother denied not paying the bill, of course, so my friend made a trip to check on her mom the next day. My friend was surprised and sad when she walked into her mother's dark house. Her mother was thin and in a panic. There were post-it notes all over the walls and furniture with reminders to herself, trying to make sense of her confusing world. The food in the refrigerator was spoiled from the electricity being turned off, and mail and other unpaid bills were stacked in piles throughout the house.

I asked my friend if she would have welcomed a call from a neighbor who likely noticed the changes in her mother. She paused for a few seconds and replied, "Of course I would." She knew the answer to her friend's question all along. Often, friends or neighbors see a person's routine change, driving skills becoming risky, or grocery shopping habits cease, but they think someone else should handle it.

That story could also be applicable to the siblings section of this chapter, but I wanted to emphasize how important neighbors can be. Please don't be afraid to visit your friend or neighbor and ask simple questions such as "I noticed you haven't been out in a while, or you just don't seem yourself, and I am concerned for you." Observe the order of the house and the cleanliness of the person and assess if they are taking care of basic needs. If you are reluctant to try this and you have family contacts, reach out or call for a welfare check. It may not be dementia, but it may be another medical need that requires attention. By becoming aware of early signs of cognitive decline, such as confusion, missing appointments, difficulty with everyday tasks, repetitive questions or conversations, or personality changes, you can play a key role in helping the person receive the services they need and deserve.

## Siblings

My two sisters and I were fortunately always on the same page when supporting our aging parents. We provided the least amount of support needed so they could feel respected and continue their lives together. If an event or circumstance called for more of our attention, we figured it out.

I was living out of town during my mother's illness, and the responsibility of providing twenty-four-hour support fell to my father and two sisters. I am so grateful to them for all the support they gave our parents, as my sister's lives were affected every day, and I carried on with mine 200 miles away. The guilt I felt was so overwhelming that I was not with my mom more often, but I struggled to even visit because of the selfish pain I felt to see her that sick.

I was working in physical rehab during this time, and when I had to go into the room of a patient on a ventilator, I began to shake and have an anxiety attack. I spoke with my supervisor and she was very understanding and adjusted my schedule to accommodate my situation. After Mom died, I left clinical permanently, realizing my strength was in behavioral health, and my weakness was in physical health.

My intense aversion to ventilators continues. I do not watch any medical shows, and I switch the channel as quickly as possible if I inadvertently scroll to a scene with a person on a ventilator. I become sick to my stomach and feel that anxiety in a matter of seconds. Ironically, my dad was placed on life support from a fall in his driveway and sustained a severe brain injury. When I arrived at the hospital, I found my sisters by his bedside, ready to comfort and reassure me, as they did eight years earlier when we lost our mother.

Two scans of my father's injury confirmed there was no brain activity. My sisters and I teamed up and made the decision to remove the life support. We were able to sing to my dad and tell stories of the good times. After the ventilator was turned off, I was holding my dad's hand when a quick tingle, almost like an electric shock, shot from my hand and out my right shoulder as he took his last breath. Instead of immediately crying, I squeezed his lifeless hand and smiled.

I also have an intense disdain when someone is so insensitive they would describe our situation as "pulling the plug." They obviously have not felt the pain and responsibility when someone's life is in your hands. I had experience working with people with traumatic brain injuries, and I knew my dad's quality of life had disappeared. You can pull the plug to remove the stopper in the sink, but you disconnect life support for someone you love because it is in the person's best interest.

Our family always made decisions together, but on that day, Dad's three girls could only speak with their voices of reason. We did not make this decision lightly but understood our dad's brain had already died. My father was not a "vegetable," a very ignorant and offensive term, but a human being, and our daddy we loved very much.

Advocating to represent and defend the rights and interests of others is a responsibility of everyone. It is not just ensuring that people or groups can live a life that is fair and just. Standing up for the rights of yourself and others who may not have a voice helps our society be more accepting and inclusive. Educating others on the unfairness of so many social issues, but when "teachable moments" present themselves, please teach.

My sisters made incredible sacrifices, especially my younger sister, as my parents began to experience health challenges. We lost my older sister during the COVID pandemic, not to the horrible virus but to the same illness my mother suffered through. So, has my family role changed from middle child to oldest sister?

If a person is diagnosed with dementia or any chronic illness and has no children or spouse to step in to assist, the responsibility for support can fall to a sibling. This was the case of a woman I recently met whose sister had early-onset Alzheimer's disease. They lived together, and the balancing act this woman does to provide care for her sister while still working is amazing. She has become well informed of the potential outcome of early onset Alzheimer's disease and is building support around her when her sister's needs become more than she is able to provide.

Brothers and sisters' experiences are different when it comes to providing care to a parent, and often, the responsibility will fall to the daughter or the daughter-in-law if the brother doesn't step up. My friend, whose mother had dementia mentioned earlier, is such an inspiration to me for the care she provided for her mom. She had a brother who lived out of state, and he was no help to her at all. He did phone his mother daily but was mostly critical of his sister regarding her care. As you may recall, he never visited his mother after she was diagnosed with Alzheimer's disease. Perhaps he felt some of my own personal struggles with my mom.

During the Christmas season, her brother confronted my friend following a phone call with his mom, questioning her why she had not put up a Christmas tree. Apparently, his mother told him they had no decorations. My friend calmly explained to her brother that not only was there a large Christmas tree in the family room but there was also a small tree in their mother's bedroom adorned with ornaments and little lights. My friend would kindly send pictures of their mother to her brother, and once he questioned why his mother's hair was so short, my friend explained to her brother that it was easier to keep her hair clean and styled.

During the late stage of Alzheimer's disease, the person may stop talking. This happened to my friend's mother, and when her mother was less able to follow the conversation with her son, he became stressed and suspicious of his sister. He thought something nefarious was going on and that she did not want him to talk to his mother.

My friend tried to explain it was part of the progression of the disease and would hold the phone to her mother's ear so he could continue speaking to his mom. Denial runs deep, as well as my admiration for my friend. She maintained her mother's quality of life until the end. I value our friendship and am grateful we stay connected. She has taught me so much about the day-to-day life and challenges of supporting a family member at home and the challenges of having a sibling who provides little support.

## LGBTQ+ Persons

After a diagnosis of dementia, LGBTQ+ persons have issues related to their identity that are different from someone who is heterosexual. These can be distressing challenges for the person and a life partner or friend when navigating the healthcare system. Karen I. Fredricksen-Goldsen, professor of Social Work at the University of Washington, states that "LGBTQ older adults are vastly underserved in most aging services and resources."

Older LGBTQ+ persons who have lived years of secrets and discrimination may not feel safe accessing healthcare services. Even in today's world, many LGTBQ+ persons are not willing to disclose their sexual orientation for fear of judgement and discrimination.

Everyone has the right to tell or not tell about their sexuality. Recently, a person with memory loss "outed" a friend in a group, not having the judgment and awareness that others in the room did not have this information. If a person with dementia has always lived a life of secrecy because of memory loss, the person might not recall who they have shared this information with and accidentally "out" themselves, making it uncomfortable for family or friends.

Because of tense relationships with parents or siblings who don't accept the person's sexual or gender identity, LGBTQ+ persons are more at risk for social isolation, which increases cognitive decline. Not only may they not have family support, they may live alone and have no children. If they do have a partner or strong social support from friends, supporting the person with dementia at home is preferred. Fear of "going back into the closet" and being treated unfairly in long-term care facilities is a real concern, and because of all the factors already mentioned, it may be their only option.

But finding an appropriate long-term placement for a friend or family member who is or isn't gay should be the same. Finding a community that meets the person's needs and interests and committing to continue advocating for your loved one offers the opportunity for a safe and engaging environment.

## Multiculturalism

Some cultural beliefs affect if and when services such as a diagnosis of dementia will be accessed. Stigma always plays a role in accepting help, and little awareness and education in some cultures are lacking. Multiple chronic illnesses and health disparities are also factors.

According to the Alzheimer's Association, Black Americans are about twice as likely to have Alzheimer's disease and other dementias than Caucasians. Hispanic Americans are more likely to have Alzheimer's disease than White Americans by about one and one-half times. Native Americans have higher rates of chronic diseases and risk factors such as diabetes, hypertension, and obesity. Some Native American languages don't even have a word for "dementia."

Dementia does not discriminate. Dementia and Alzheimer's disease affect people of all genders, races, sexes, races, and ethnicities. Assuming everyone fits in neat little boxes will promote stereotypes and create barriers to healthcare services.

I recognize I am not doing justice by not going into more detail on the effects culture, race, ethnicity, and even gender have on the social issue, perception, stigma, and most importantly, the discrimination of our society for quality healthcare, and I do apologize. These issues most definitely and urgently need to be addressed, as well as so many other social issues and basic human rights that affect our neighbors, friends, or even ourselves, that make life an uphill battle to achieving one's full potential. It is not my lack of commitment to expound on these global issues because creating an inclusive, equal, and diverse society matters and is, at my core, part of my identity. But this is not the time nor place. But if you join me and others in advocating for the rights of all those living with dementia or Alzheimer's disease, you can make a difference, if only for one person.

## Person Living with Dementia

During an expressive art class for persons living with memory loss, the activity was to draw a self-portrait. One gentleman drew an apple tree to the left of his paper with a dark blue cloud overhead. To the right of the tree, he drew a man with a smile and a bright yellow shirt. He was holding one purple balloon and was drifting up toward a bright yellow sun in the sky. When I asked him to tell me about the picture, he replied, "I sometimes feel like I'm floating." Such a profound statement he was able to express through art.

People living with dementia often experience sudden changes in their emotional responses and, due to the neurological changes in the brain, have less control over their emotions with communication challenges and have difficulty expressing those feelings. A person may misinterpret a kind touch as a sexual expression. Or misunderstand a comment and think someone is making fun of them.

Some people who live with cognitive decline, even in the later progression of memory loss, are aware of their lapses in memory, difficulty finding words, and confusion. One man described it as "drifting" through the stages. However, many do not recognize or have any awareness of their behaviors, troubling comments, or actions and may be experiencing agnosia, the inability to recognize or acknowledge their cognitive impairment.

This phenomenon is difficult for the person and their family member and friends. Since the person does not recognize that perhaps he/she is no longer safe to drive, cook, or handle their finances, trying to convince them only creates major conflicts. When someone does not know their limitations, reckless and dangerous behaviors can jeopardize the safety and well-being of the person and others. Agnosia complicates the treatment approach, and the person will need to rely on you or someone else for healthcare and medical decision-making.

Listening and observing the feelings can offer insight into the frustration of being unable to complete a familiar task. Validating the frustration and "stretching the truth" about certain concerns can help. Be mindful of offering help when you see it is needed, but if your family member refuses, allow them to accomplish the task, even though it is not done perfectly.

## Self

Would identifying as a "caregiver" cloud your judgment when the needs of your friend or loved one become more than your skills? Would you continue giving care regardless of your own health or the safety of the person? Are you a caregiver, or are you still a wife, daughter, mother, sibling, husband, sister, or son who provides care, and thus, you can make decisions in the best interest of your loved one?

Imagine if you were in their position. Imagine that your spouse, son, daughter, sibling, or friend suddenly takes control of your life and tells you the things you can and cannot do, eat or drink, or who you can talk to see. Imagine not feeling respected, valued, or never given choices again. Each family is different when a dementia diagnosis comes knocking on the door. Relationship dynamics prior to the diagnosis, the family's understanding of dementia, the type of dementia, and the emotional capacity of family members all play into understanding the diagnosis and influence how the family opens the door. Ideally, this unexpected, unwanted, and intrusive visitor will be greeted by the whole family. Not necessarily with open arms and a warm welcome, but by answering the door together, the family is better equipped to navigate and understand the challenges dementia may bring. Family members can also have a clearer perspective of the importance of self-care so the person will receive the best care possible.

It is impossible to address every relationship, role, or culture that impacts the care of a person living with a neurocognitive disorder. The employer, the co-worker, the aunt, the niece, and the list goes on. But hopefully, you will begin to see where your role fits in the person's life and the influence you could have on their care, well-being, and future outcomes. This chapter is just snippets of examples of the roles we play in life and the importance of knowing that what you do is not who you are.

## Activity 1

Imagine your spouse, son, or daughter suddenly taking control of your life. This requires telling you the things you can and cannot do, where and when you go somewhere, and who you can and cannot socialize with. They would also control what you eat, the activities you offer, or how your money is spent. Imagine you don't feel respected or valued and were never given choices again.

Use the space below to express how that would make you feel and respond.

## Activity 2

Self-awareness creates growth and a better understanding of ourselves. Feeling powerlessness, the anxiety can create a strong desire to control situations, circumstances, and people you care for may not feel safe. It may be unconscious,' but it helps us to maintain a sense of order in our lives. Do you use the "take charge" or "my way or the highway" approach in your life? How can this approach affect the relationship with a family member living with dementia?

Use the space below to explore times when perhaps a softer and less authoritarian approach might have worked better.

# Chapter 7
## Self Efficacy

*"I think I can, I think I can, I think I can!"* -The Little Engine That Could

In the classic children's book, *The Little Engine That Could*, a small blue locomotive with no experience pulling long trains came to the rescue of a big red train that broke down and was unable to finish its journey over a large mountain to deliver toys to the children. The little blue locomotive not only had no experience pulling such a large train, but she had never even crossed over the big mountain.

Bigger trains did not want to help the big red train, but the little blue engine volunteered because she knew the children were expecting the toys. She huffed and puffed as she began the steep climb up the mountain, chanting, "I think I can, I think I can, I think I can!" pulling the big red train behind. The little blue engine struggled as she neared the top but continued repeating, "I think I can, I think I can."

As the cadence of her words became faster, the speed of the little blue engine increased, and she successfully crossed over the mountain with the big red engine in tow. This was only possible because the little blue engine believed she could cross that mountain. This simple short story is a perfect example of psychologist Albert Bandura's theory of self-efficacy; "A person's particular set of beliefs that determine how well one can execute a plan of action in prospective situations" (Bandura, 1977). To put it in simpler terms, self-efficacy is a person's belief in their ability to succeed in a particular situation.

Referring to an earlier reference in the book on the effectiveness of positive "self-talk," Bandura believed, as do I, motivational self-talk significantly increases not only self-efficacy but also the performance of the task. People with a strong sense of efficacy or a strong belief in themselves are more likely to tackle difficult challenges and overcome setbacks quickly.

Mastery of a skill is essential when developing a strong belief in yourself. By building on personal experiences and existing skills, the success ratio in the future is more likely. The Learning Zone Model, developed by psychologist Lev Vygotsky, can be a start in overcoming perceived challenges. This model encourages stepping out of your comfort zone and taking small risks to learn something new. The idea is that the more you move out of your comfort zone, or the place where every skill is easy and almost second nature, to a risk-taking zone, the feelings of fear and dread, the fear of taking risks will lessen, and the new skills can be mastered. This will also have a positive effect on self-esteem or how we feel about ourselves overall.

For instance, stepping out of our comfort zone, exposing ourselves to risks, and possibly exposing our vulnerabilities results in personal growth. Taking an online class, joining a hobby club, testing the waters, and trying new skills in this book can lead to higher self-efficacy and make other risks less scary.

Teaching self-efficacy and helping someone believe in themselves is probably the most rewarding part of my profession. Working with individuals with many types of disabilities and learning to believe in themselves is key to accomplishing something hard. For example, teaching children with intellectual disabilities to believe in themselves is essential when learning skills such as riding a bicycle, independently putting on a backpack for a hike, or developing social skills to not only make friends but how to keep them. By teaching family members self-efficacy skills and the importance of believing in themselves, families are better equipped to help their loved one with dementia believe in themselves and can promote independence as long as possible.

Bandura's theory also suggests that self-efficacy is seen as a stress-coping strategy. By developing high self-efficacy or beliefs, you have more control of your life with skills to regulate stress, and your confidence to handle stressors and reduce episodes of panic or making mistakes will decrease. Self-esteem can influence confidence, trust, and belief in our self-efficacy and can influence motivation to learn new skills. Changing our attitudes toward a circumstance, person, or belief can be difficult but possible. Exploring our attitudes and values and identifying the source of an attitude or a limiting belief about ourselves is the beginning of changing a negative belief into a positive belief. We only incorporate those beliefs we value into our lives.

People with low self-efficacy avoid tasks that seem challenging and often perceive difficult tasks and circumstances as beyond existing capabilities. People with low self-efficacy will also avoid learning new skills, focusing on their weaknesses rather than strengths and are quickly discouraged and lose belief in their possible potential.

On the other hand, people with high self-efficacy will approach new challenges with confidence and gusto. When you believe in yourself, you can dive deeper into self-awareness and gain a better understanding of your needs as well as your loved ones. Developing resilience will allow you to bounce back quicker from a negative experience. By embracing the L.O.V.E. Approach and practicing listening, observing, validating, and engaging with your loved one, problem-solving becomes easier. You can approach new challenges with commitment and feelings of accomplishment.

Why is high self-efficacy useful in supporting someone with dementia? Research shows that people living with dementia will generally need more support from their family members than people with other chronic illnesses. (Pinquart& Sorensen, 2003; Spector & Kemper, 1994) The National Library of Medicine, the world's largest medical library, published a study indicating that "self-efficacy training, an in-depth understanding of dementia behavior symptoms and psychosocial interventions" can determine a more positive experience for families when supporting someone at home. Because of the physical requirements, emotional stress, behavioral symptoms, communication challenges, and cognitive decline that come when caring for someone with dementia, the person providing care can have serious negative health consequences known as "caregiver burden."

The term "burden" can be confusing when referring to caregiving. I recently received a call from the son of a gentleman I have been working with. The son was upset and very angry. He and his father had just returned home from an appointment with his father's neurologist. It was confirmed his dad did have Alzheimer's disease. However, the diagnosis wasn't unexpected, and the family had already been using the L.O.V.E. Approach in supporting the father.

Apparently, the doctor attempted to explain to the son the negative consequences of caregiving and the "burden of care." The burden of care is the perceived stress when caring for someone and is one of the most important warnings for the possible negative health outcomes of those providing care, especially when caring for someone with dementia. The son misinterpreted his comment and flatly denied his father was a "burden."

When I explained what the doctor tried to convey and reassured the son our coaching sessions were developing strategies to reduce the "burden of care" by developing self-efficacy skills, he immediately calmed down. Research shows that family members with high self-efficacy who care for someone with cognitive decline "experience lower burden and depressive symptom severity."

Because of the progression of dementia, the length of time supporting someone at home varies, and family members are at risk for depression and anxiety. Females providing constant care may also be less likely to get regular screenings (such as a depression screening), and they may not get enough sleep or regular physical activity. American Psychological Association. (2012). Stress in America: Our Health at Risk. APA: Washington, DC. I was facilitating a workshop, and when this topic was being discussed, one woman who cares for her husband with dementia started shaking her head and shared that she was a cancer survivor and had rescheduled her annual screening three times, stretching the screening to almost two years. She committed then to making the next screening a priority.

**Women caring for a spouse are more likely to have high blood pressure, diabetes, and high cholesterol and are twice as likely to have heart disease. (14)**

Stress can be sneaky and suddenly appear, causing anger, frustration, or even confusion. Mistakes when giving medication or forgetting an important appointment are common when stress is not managed well. Being overwhelmed and feeling tired most of the time can affect decision-making skills, which can result in becoming more stressed. The ability to make good decisions directly influences our ability to make progress.

Attitudes and behaviors are connected to our emotional pain from a past distressing event(s) that may be holding us back from having the ability to move forward and look at our circumstances differently. Many core beliefs stem from our childhood, parents, and early life experiences. By understanding how a negative belief or attitude was formed, shifting to a positive and more useful belief, reducing negative thought patterns, and practicing positive self-talk, positive change can be achieved.

Do you believe in your ability to complete difficult tasks? Do you have the confidence to learn and master new skills that may require great effort to achieve a goal? What holds you back from making a positive change? Trusting in yourself and having faith that you can influence your environment impacts the care and support you provide to your loved one and helps to maintain your motivation and well-being.

Motivation? Are you kidding me? With all the responsibility of providing constant support, you now want me to maintain my motivation too? According to Teresa Amabile and Steven Kramer in their 2011 book, *The Progress Principle*, there is nothing more motivating than progress. Even the smallest of consistent achievements can "significantly boost people's motivation and performance."

Self-efficacy can be achieved with the mastery of skills (practicing the new skill until it is learned). Thus, the feeling of competence and confidence will develop. Little successes help to build emotional resilience and lead to self-determination, or the ability to be in control of decisions and make choices that influence our lives without outside influence. Like self-efficacy, self-determination is a process with highs and lows as you begin to trust yourself more and are willing to stand up to those who are trying to force you to meet their expectations.

So, what is the difference between self-determination and self-efficacy? Self-efficacy is the belief that you can learn new skills and provide quality care for your family member or friend, and self-determination focuses on your ability to make your own decisions and choices based on your values and goals. The more understanding and awareness you have about the symptoms of dementia, the more able you are to try new strategies to decrease dementia-related behaviors of your loved one, and the more you believe in yourself to make informed decisions regarding care.

I specialize in personal phone coaching to teach self-efficacy to family members supporting someone with dementia. Studies show that this approach, along with motivational interviewing (a technique to help people find the motivation to make positive behavioral changes), is effective in increasing self-efficacy and can be maintained over time.

When coaching families, it is not unusual to observe the unintentional disregard adult children or other relatives can have toward the significance of a parents' long-time relationship and take away the ability for the parents to maintain self-determination. Because of the younger ages of the adult child, or perhaps even the reality, they have not experienced a long-term relationship with a spouse or partner, dismissing the significance of the companionship their parents shared for many years, perhaps seventy years or more, can become problematic.

I was coaching a husband whose wife had recently transitioned to a memory care community after caring for her at home for ten years. Sadly, his two daughters lack the empathy and compassion to support him during this time and continue to tell him to "Move on. Mom is safe." Safety has nothing to do with the loneliness and sadness their father is living now. Ironically, both daughters have experienced divorces and may lack the understanding of the impact loss of a long-term relationship has on grief.

Although his wife is still living, he is grieving the loss of their relationship. His grief is personal and his own and should be respected and supported. Moving someone into memory care may relieve the adult children of responsibilities, but it is a new level of grief for the spouse, and the responsibilities have not ended. Expecting someone to "move on" during the grief process is not only unhelpful, it is hurtful.

For the most part, adult children want what is best for their parents, but leaping from the "facts" of the situation and disregarding the "feelings" of the parent without dementia can cause significant consequences for that parent. Whether it is a forced or voluntary move to a new city or transitioning a parent into a memory care community, not acknowledging and validating the pain, fear, and loneliness the parent without dementia is experiencing, depression, reduction in quality of life, and even cognitive decline can occur.

Focusing on someone else's needs and neglecting our own can affect how we feel about ourselves. We can become detached from our feelings, thoughts, and beliefs and become absorbed in work, alcohol, food, or electronics. We fail to recognize our feelings and needs. When we neglect our needs, our self-image can change as well, and we may become ashamed of how tired we look. A study showed that people who care for someone with dementia become distressed when "neglecting their health and well-being as their energies and efforts are directed to the person receiving care."

With the progression of dementia, the person must depend on others to assist with everyday tasks and encourage engagement. The nebulous concept of improving quality of life is baffling when you are unable to recognize your own personal needs because the focus is on providing excellent care for your loved one. This makes you increasingly susceptible to health problems. If you become ill, have an emergency, or just burn out, it may be difficult to ask for help. Even so, reaching out to others is necessary in order to keep both you and your loved one healthy and safe.

When we become stumped because interactions become stressful, friends and even family members may disappear. This can leave the primary support family member and the person with dementia feeling abandoned and alone. Imagine if you received a cancer diagnosis and everyone just vanished. Spending time with your friend or loved one can bring joy and create moments that will matter and lead to positive memories to cherish. Is there currently someone in your life living with dementia or caring for that person you could call today and offer your support and understanding?

Planning and creating preventative measures to stay healthy can be challenging, but it is worth doing. Taking time to get away when able, participating in an enjoyable hobby, fulfilling social and physical/exercise needs, and filling up spiritually all result in a greater sense of well-being and happiness. Keep your health in check first so you can be there for your loved one in the ways that you wish. Using the airplane analogy "should an emergency occur" and placing your oxygen mask on first when traveling with a child says it all. If you run out of oxygen, you obviously can't help anyone else. This may sound selfish, but please give yourself permission to take care of your own needs and avoid running out of air.

Can you start today and give yourself permission to take care of your needs so you can feel more refreshed tomorrow? Are you ready to look at yourself with a more objective eye? Are you willing to make little changes in your approach when speaking to your loved one to help them feel less shame and embarrassment in the future?

Are you ready to try a new approach for supporting your loved one or friend that could possibly create a healthier relationship for both of you? Can you begin to find shared moments of joy and create more happiness in your life?

Research shows the relationship between self-efficacy and happiness is strongly connected. Studies also show that people with high self-efficacy are happier people, and happier people can achieve self-efficacy more easily. Can you begin to think of ideas to engage your loved one, share in joyful experiences, and create more happiness in your home?

I am generally a pretty happy and optimistic person, and it has been suggested I possibly see the world "through rose-colored glasses," expecting the best outcomes. People who see life with greater objectivity may balk at this approach, believing this is unrealistic and that negative aspects of life are ignored. Research, however, shows just the opposite and seeing life "through rose-colored glasses" can literally make everything seem a bit more vibrant and clear. Viewing the world in a more positive light can help expand your awareness and your ability to appreciate the small things in your life.

Self-efficacy is a process. We may have high self-efficacy in one area and low self-efficacy in another, but overall, it is how we value ourselves and internalize the meaning of our identity. Executing the strategies to listen, observe, validate, and engage with your loved one or friend will help you bounce back quicker from stressful situations, be more hopeful in making thoughtful decisions, find solutions to new challenges, and increase your self-confidence. You will be more prepared for unexpected events and stay calm during difficult situations. You will achieve and recognize the small successes and maintain the motivation to keep going.

Just like the little blue engine who believed in herself and started her descent from the top of the mountain chanting, "I thought I could, I thought I could, I thought I could," believe in yourself the next time you are faced with a difficult task or decision. What you choose to believe about yourself is one of the most consequential decisions you make.

Never let your fears stop you from trying something new and making changes in your life. Another great icon of Tennessee and a great love of mine, Dolly Parton, believes, "You'll never do a whole lot unless you're brave enough to try." As a child, I related so well with the Cowardly Lion in The Wizard of Oz and loved the way he would settle his nerves by stroking his tail. Much like the Cowardly Lion, I conquered great feats of bravery by doing hard things growing up. It takes courage to change, and it isn't always easy. But it is possible once you realize the need to change.

### (Singing)

*I'm afraid there's no denyin'*
*I'm just a dandy lion*
*A fate I don't deserve*

*I'm sure I could show my prowess*
*Be a lion, not a mouse*
*If I only had the nerve*

*-The Cowardly Lion from The Wizard of OZ*

## Activity 1

Self-efficacy: Identify the skills that are hard when supporting your loved one and the possible reasons they may seem difficult. (Unresolved relationship issues, feelings of inadequacy)

## Activity 2

Looking at Activity 1 above, identify ways to find the courage to increase your belief in yourself and increase your self-efficacy.

## Activity 3

Stop "shoulding" on yourself! For instance, identify the negative self-talk you tell yourself, such as:

- "I should know how to do this."
- "I should be more patient."
- " I should have known this would make him mad."
- 
- 
- 

## Activity 4

Replace your negative self-talk with positive self-talk, such as:

- " This is hard, but with practice, I can be more patient."
- "I've never done this before, but I believe I can master this!"
- 
- 
- 
- 
- 
-

## Chapter 8
## A Need for Change

As mentioned in the first chapter, after Pat Summit announced her diagnosis of early-onset Alzheimer's in 2011, my career took an unexpected turn. Pat fought for causes much of her life, such as changing the world of women's sports, fighting for pay equality for collegiate coaches, and even fighting off a raccoon once to save her dog, which dislocated her shoulder, to name a few. She fought with courage and tenacity, and the fight against this new opponent, dementia, was no different.

I understood the stigma a diagnosis brings, and her decision to fight this disease publicly honestly gave me hope that the stigma of dementia could change. It was only two months earlier Glen Campbell had gone public with his diagnosis of Alzheimer's disease, and I felt this might be a turning point to de-stigmatize the perceptions of dementia.

Pat was a mother, sister, daughter, aunt, cousin, and friend, and I immediately felt an insatiable desire to learn as much as I could about how dementia affects the well-being and emotional health of family and friends who love someone living with dementia. I am certainly not trying to tell Pat's story but the overwhelming support from her family, coaches, Lady Vols, and thousands of aspiring young athletes across the nation who rallied around her with love and support, joining the "We Back Pat" campaign, gave me pause.

When I first began researching articles and books available to families on dementia care, my first observation was how often a negative metaphor was used in the title. I found several guides on how to "survive" or "cope" and the "challenges" of caring for someone with dementia can bring. One even recommended strategies to survive a "land mine."

Other metaphors compared dementia to a "ticking time bomb" and to natural disasters such as tsunamis, storms, or floods. Several even described the person with dementia as "vanishing" or "disappearing" as if they no longer exist, and a couple of books compared dementia to a "monster" to be feared. The most astounding book title for me was the idea that "caregivers" would be providing not just 24-hour care but an additional 12 hours in one day. That sounds pretty overwhelming.

With the heightened emotions of anxiety and trepidation family members and friends feel, and dementia is suspected, the fear can be profuse. Imagine starting your research like I did and finding book titles that are frightening but ironically were intended to change your attitudes and strategies to address dementia. Fear-based messaging generally does not work to promote long-term behavioral changes.

In the 1970's, the New Jersey Scared Straight Program was created as a fear-based approach to prevent juvenile delinquency. However, a randomized trail was conducted and concluded the program had no effect on changing behaviors of those who went through the program.

As a young therapist working in addiction during this time, one job responsibility I was charged I absolutely abhorred was taking teenagers from the treatment facility to the local prison to hear inmates attempt to "scare them straight" into behaving in hopes prison would not be their life's outcome. I was terrified in the beginning and recall young twelve, thirteen even seventeen-year-old boys crying, one throwing up on my shoe as we were leaving once.

On a side note, during one visit, a prisoner who regularly spoke in the presentations presented me an ink drawing he had done in appreciation for letting him tell his story to "my kids." I was grateful this experience did have a positive effect on at least one prisoner I befriended.

Words influence the ways we think, feel, make decisions and even how we treat people. The words dementia and Alzheimer's alone evoke fear in people because of the long history of negative misinformation. Evoking more fear in people who are committed to supporting a person with dementia by using scary language doesn't make sense to me. We may not realize the impact negative words can have on our attitudes and perceptions, which can lead to feelings of a "hopeless situation" for the family. This will result in low expectations of the person living with dementia and limit the capacity for the person to live a life with purpose and quality for a longer period of time.

Various resources are important and necessary for families, and I am not suggesting these books do not have valuable and helpful information. But words are powerful and can influence the perception of how we see and understand dementia. Words can empower you or discourage you. The language used to describe dementia as someone who is "suffering," "afflicted," "an empty shell," "victim," "demented, "senile," or "not being all there," and the most disrespectful, insensitive, and derogatory description of a person living with dementia as being "a vegetable," only perpetuates the stigma, distress and discrimination that can delay treatment. Negative language can cause doubt and despair for the family, but imagine the fear a person experiencing cognitive concerns feels when they begin randomly looking for books online or browsing through a bookstore to understand what is happening to them and come across books with negative messaging like I did.

Utilizing a strengths-based approach to dementia care (what your loved one can do rather than what they can't do) and taking time to explain your loved one has a medical condition that affects memory, thinking skills, and judgment, and with positive interactions and patience, the person can continue to remain independent longer may make dementia less scary. Advocating for your family member or friend and believing you and your loved one can live with dementia together encourages others to engage and continue to share meaningful connections.

Using respectful language when speaking of someone living with dementia not only helps to honor their dignity but also promotes an awareness that a diagnosis of dementia does not define the person. Dementia does not take away a person's dignity. People do. There are many types of dementia, and each person is a unique individual. When you have met one person with dementia, you have met one person with dementia, just as if you met one athlete, you have met one athlete because everyone is different. We all have our individual personalities, likes and dislikes, preferences and needs, and dementia affects each individual differently.

The person does not cease to be who they are or change from an adult into a "child," and they are definitely not "an empty shell." It is our responsibility to learn and practice how to connect with the person where they are and do things with the person, not for the person to promote independence, self-worth and dignity. Concluding that all people with dementia are the same reinforces the stereotypes and stigma dementia brings, and a diagnosis of dementia does not reflect the person's level of ability to understand.

Fortunately, newer authors and newer book titles are evolving and seem to recognize the need to present a more hopeful outcome and de-stigmatize the hopeless perceptions many have of dementia. This is important as it can help raise awareness, dispel the myths about dementia, and encourage others to use more appropriate language and informed awareness, thus helping to shift the paradigm of dementia's perception. Titles with words such as "joy," "meaningful," and "living" seem much more encouraging than "coping," "managing," or "surviving" a medical condition your loved one is living with every day.

After my disappointment in the less-than-optimistic book titles and questionable language used to help "caregivers," I felt I needed more first-hand understanding of the messages the professional community was sending families. I continued my quest and attended in-person and online training. I wanted to learn from the established professionals what family members were hearing, seeing, and doing in the training and the treatment approach professionals were sharing, specifically for those supporting someone in the home. Sadly, again, I was disillusioned by what I discovered.

I wasn't sure what to expect from the training or the specific information to be taught. However, being a trainer and group facilitator for over forty years, I supposed I did have a preconceived notion the training would be based on adult learning theories, evidence-based interventions, experiential and hands-on experiences, small discussion groups, and a process or debriefing session at the conclusion.

Unfortunately, that is not what I found. Most trainings used a classroom style approach with PowerPoint presentations filled with paragraphs, bullet points, statistics and images of a compromised or dying brain. Many of the training began with this image using clinical terms identifying parts of the brain and the effects on memory, reasoning, language, social skills and so on.

This is helpful information because it is important to understand how a person with dementia experiences symptoms. However, it was very intense, and even as a healthcare professional who understands neurocognitive disorders, it was overwhelming. I don't know if perhaps presenting this information in smaller segments with breaks would make it less intimidating, or perhaps it was just me because, with each word spoken in the training, I was watching and imaging how family members felt as they tried to relate this information to their family member, a person, not just a brain.

I was very surprised by the lack of distinction for the suitability for whom the training targeted. Two of the in-person trainings I attended included healthcare staff and family members. Healthcare professionals and families have different needs as well as different abilities to process information; thus, combining these groups didn't seem logical to me. Repeated clinical terms are appropriate for healthcare staff; however, it may be very confusing and could be beyond some family member's ability to relate the information for practical purposes.

My biggest concern, however, was some family members brought their loved ones with dementia to the training. Subjecting someone living with dementia to an event that is discussing topics they are unable to process accurately is never appropriate, in my professional opinion. When I questioned a trainer from a national organization regarding the inclusion of people with dementia in a training designed for "caregivers," she reasoned families have trouble finding respite care and "there are not that many that attend."

I believe one person is too many. The training addresses such sensitive issues, and although people living with dementia experience confusion and memory difficulties in the early stages, they can still feel shame and fear and are very aware when they are being talked about. Disregarding the vulnerability and the need to respect the dignity of someone living with dementia by exposing them to information they are unable to process does not seem ethical.

Allowing a person with dementia to attend a training designed for family members also enables the families to not ask for help. Reaching out to other family members, friends, or neighbors and inviting them to visit with your loved one while the family member attends the training can be a good option. Asking for help is difficult; however, it can delay a family from exploring other options for assistance, such as a home health agency a couple of days a week for respite. It is always best to identify resources before you need them and not allow an incident to make a decision for you.

My commitment to supporting the dignity and respect of someone living with dementia is steadfast, runs deep in my soul, and will not be compromised. When someone registers for my training, I follow up with a phone call to ensure their family member will be safe and taken care of so they attend. If I am told there is no one to care for their family member, I provide guidance and help the family explore possible solutions. I have had very few families that did not somehow find care for their family members and were able to attend that training, and I often see them in the next one.

I don't fault the families as they often feel they have such few options. It is hard for me to wrap my mind around the inability of organizations that raise and spend billions of dollars to find a cure and develop pharmacological interventions but miss the mark to provide respite services during a training so family members can receive support.

During a local in-person training I attended, a woman questioned the newest Alzheimer's drug. The trainer answered rather emphatically that to be aware it only treats symptoms because there is no cure for Alzheimer's disease. The man sitting beside her became restless. My guess was he was her husband and perhaps had early-stage Alzheimer's disease and became frightened by this news, which he likely had heard before but forgotten.

I saw the couple and the trainer speaking afterward and overhead the trainer making amends for her abrupt blunder. In this same training, a man and wife sitting behind me also had an unfortunate incident. The topic was how to "deal" with apathy, and the woman pointed to her husband and jokingly asked the presenter, "How can I get him to do anything but watch TV?". The audience responded with an uncomfortable chuckle, and I saw that all-too-familiar look of shame and tears in the gentleman's eyes.

I also took a 12-hour virtual evidence-based training broken into 2-hour weekly sessions. The trainer was knowledgeable and compassionate, and the group developed a comforting bond. The trainer knew I was also a dementia trainer and welcomed me to the group. The sessions flowed well and covered a variety of helpful topics. This training was originally developed in 2002, and one video was outdated.

The professional in the video was demonstrating a prompting technique with a woman with dementia. They were making a ham and cheese sandwich, and unintentionally, the professional embarrassed the woman by pointing out that she did not "remember" to put the ham on first. Family members likely didn't even notice, but my ability to find four-leaf clovers, catch bloopers in movies and observe the smallest details are both a blessing and a curse.

During another training I attended, the facilitator explained inappropriate social behaviors that may occur when someone with cognitive decline has lost inhibitions and judgment due to changes in the brain. I was stunned when the trainer grabbed and held her crouch area for a few seconds and began mimicking a mumbling and confused woman (or perhaps a man), shaking her head, holding her mouth open with a protruding tongue and exaggerated, distorted facial expressions.

As the trainer was demonstrating this inappropriate social behavior of someone who has lost control of thinking and reasoning that can cause embarrassing situations, I wondered if any thought was given to the inappropriate behavior of the trainer. I quickly surveyed the room and heard the uncomfortable but familiar laughter from many of the professional healthcare staff who perhaps saw this demonstration as entertaining. Still, when I looked at the family members in the audience, many had a blank stare, and I think they were as shocked as I was. Perhaps this was an isolated incident, but mimicry of someone with a disability is never cute or appropriate and using humor at the expense of someone with a disability is incredibly insensitive.

People living with dementia must always be respected to maintain their dignity and not be made to feel any less than a human being. Humor, laughter and playfulness are effective strategies to connect emotionally with people, and I use them often to "promote a healthy, safe and healing environment" (31), but like tasteless jokes, making people laugh at the expense of certain groups delivers a negative hidden message.

But as unsettling as this incident was, it was the "and then moment." "The ah-ha second," and the sudden flipped switch of the giant bulb lighting up my brain. My eyes opened wide from the glare of that metaphorical illumination, and by coming out of the darkness, I realized change was needed in supporting family members and friends who care for a loved one living with dementia: these families deserve a new approach to training and resources to meet their specific needs. A sudden burst of inspiration overcame me, and it was that moment I decided to begin the fight for the need to pay more attention to the symptoms of dementia in the family members, not just their loved ones.

The word "fight" can have a negative connotation, as if dementia is a war and not a medical condition to be treated. But it is what it is. We certainly cannot just disagree, squabble, dispute or fuss about dementia. We must all fight not just for a cure but for a more balanced and integrated holistic, humanistic, whole-body, family-centered and eco-psychosocial approach to treating families and their loved one.

As I was sitting in that training, surrounded by family members and friends who loved someone living with dementia, I could see the pain in their faces and bodies and feel the fear as I watched the information sink in and the glum and hopeless looks displayed as if perhaps they were watching a movie of a dismal future for their family. Were they also having an "and then moment" and realizing how overwhelming "caregiving" will be? I thought of Coach Summitt and her fierce determination to fight and advocate for herself and her commitment and desire to remain coaching and showing such courage to coach "as long as the good Lord is willing". With accommodations and additional support from her staff, she was given the opportunity to continue living with purpose and passion, leading her team to win her final SEC Tournament Championship in 2012 before retiring.

Studies suggest that family "caregivers" for people with dementia are often considered "invisible patients" for neglecting their own health and well-being and the sacrifices made. The social isolation they experience can result in depression, and the financial concerns and day-to-day responsibilities can make family members physically and emotionally sick. Because it affects every member of the family, it was puzzling to me that training does not adequately address the serious health issues family members can develop other than promoting self-care and support groups. So I began researching what "family caregivers" really need, and the L.O.V.E. Approach was born.

This chapter, or perhaps even the book, may spark criticism and even controversy, but the late John Lewis, who devoted his life to racial inequalities, said, "Never, ever be afraid to make some noise and get in good trouble, necessary trouble." Like Mr. Lewis, I have never been afraid to speak the truth and will always be honest. My convictions and beliefs in this book are solely based on my research, education, professional and personal life experiences, values, and ongoing efforts to promote and foster equity, diversity and inclusion for everyone, especially those living with dementia and their families and friends.

## Activity 1

Change is always difficult. If you make changes, what do you think will work for you and your family? Please use the space below to identify the strengths you have to make those changes.

## Activity 2

What worries you the most about your current situation? What would be the advantage of making changes to address some of your concerns? Please use the space below to brainstorm ideas.

Activity 3

Do you have your own health concerns and is something stopping you from making changes to address these concerns? Are you prepared for the consequences of not addressing these concerns? Please answer below.

## Chapter 9
## Living with Purpose and Meaning

*"Love life. Engage in it. Give it all you've got. Love it with a passion because life truly does give back, many times over, what you put into it."* — Maya Angelou

Our purpose in life changes throughout our lifespan and is not bounded by just one purpose. We can have many purposes that encompass different areas of our lives. Living with purpose brings meaning into each day, and like happiness, purpose is not a destination to be sought but rather part of the journey of living a fulfilled life. Having purpose reflects on our ever-changing goals and the desire to pursue them.

Roles in our lives can change as well. When people provide care for someone with a disability or declining health and find themselves in a "caregiving role," the negative aspects of caregiving seem to dominate the vision of what caregiving actually is. In a review of positive aspects of caregiving, four main domains were identified: "a sense of personal accomplishment and gratification, feelings of mutuality in a dyadic relationship, an increase of family cohesion and functionality, and a sense of personal growth and purpose in life." (15)

Sound familiar? The foundation of the L.O.V.E. Approach does just that: teaching self-efficacy and self-determine skills to promote a sense of confidence and acknowledgment of accomplishments, sharing in meaningful activities and creating mutual relationships. Using a family-centered treatment approach, avoiding an imbalance of power, and gaining self-awareness resulting in personal growth and one's purpose in life, creates well-being is the essence of this approach.

Personal growth by seeking to "know one's self" helps us see and understand our world and live a life of well-being and purpose. Even the smallest gestures can contribute to our well-being. A recent Gallup poll found that adults who "regularly say hello to their neighbors" have a higher sense of well-being than those who do not, and people with purpose have better health and are generally happier people. While meaning and purpose are personal and about our "being," identifying goals that align with our purpose is more specific and requires "action." When we lack purpose, we feel lost with little direction in our lives.

As we age and begin thinking about retirement, many people will take the opportunity to experience a renewed sense of purpose in life. There are many factors related to the decision to retire or to continue working. According to research, most people look forward to retirement and live with more freedom and spend more time with family. However, when someone retires unwillingly due to health concerns or is forced out of a work setting due to downsizing or other reasons with no fault of their own, they are often not prepared for the abundance of "free time."

With limited financial resources and a lack of leisure interests, many new retirees flounder aimlessly or return to the workforce, perhaps part-time. Our social, physical, cognitive, expressive and often, spiritual needs are met in our work settings by nature, and without preparation to address these needs outside of work in retirement, the person is at risk of social isolation, depression, and decreased well-being, and feeling a loss of purpose in their life. Healthcare professionals recognize for some people, retirement can have a negative influence on the person's health, not just for the person but also for the family.

I work with older adults in several capacities and teach a retirement planning class focusing on leisure skills, leisure education, leisure planning, time management and personal and community resources, "Are You Ready for 25 Years of Free Time?" People's retirement plans will include financial strategies, downsizing, and even moving closer to family, but seldom do I come across someone who takes a close look at the significance of ensuring their social, physical, cognitive and expressive needs are met through a balance of hobbies and pursuing interests that will help facilitate a healthy adjustment to retirement and continue to live a meaningful and purposeful life. Leisure alone does not improve quality of life. You must know how to use it.

I had rotator cuff surgery this past summer (the other shoulder, not the one from the bird attack) and was waiting for my physical therapy appointment. There were several people in the waiting room, some in my age group and a few bit older. A woman, perhaps in her early 70's with a walker, noticed my sling and asked what happened. I told her and then asked about her swollen knee. She explained since she retired, she has just "gone downhill." This started a spontaneous and lively conversation, and this conjecture was the consensus of the group. Retirement transitions can be difficult if you are not prepared to continue and maintain an active life you enjoyed during your working years. Poor health, falls, and depression in retirement are just a few of the consequences of neglecting your social, physical, cognitive, expressive and spiritual needs throughout your life. Recreation is an essential element of human biology, both mentally and physically.

Stuart Brown, M.D. details in his book *Play: How it Shapes the Brain*, Opens the Imagination, and Invigorates the Soul, defines play as "apparently purposeless activity (done for its own sake), voluntary, inherent attraction, freedom from time, diminished consciousness of self, improvisational potential, and continuation desire." and suggests that play and recreation are necessary for a "full and flourishing life."

*"People who cannot find time for recreation are obliged sooner or later to find time for illness."*
-John Wanamaker.

Declining health will impact when and why someone may retire, this includes the health of the retiree, as well as the family members. One study found "women are five times more likely to retire to care for a family member." But men are not excluded from falling into a caregiving role. It is estimated that 40% of family caregivers are men.

So what if you are living with a neurocognitive disorder such as dementia or Alzheimer's disease? How does that affect one's purpose, meaning and quality of life? Studies show that with dementia, a person's sense of purpose can decline, not just after the diagnosis but also leading up to the diagnosis. You may have noticed, perhaps a year or two prior to the diagnosis, that your loved one's motivational level and zest for life lessened. However, living with dementia does not mean purpose is not important or possible to achieve. With support, people living with dementia can continue to live with purpose and meaning in their lives despite cognitive decline, even during later stages, with the support of the family.

With that in mind, consider possible changes in your sense of purpose since your loved one began showing signs of cognitive decline or memory loss. When the changes in the brain begin to interfere with difficult tasks, activities of daily living (dressing, hygiene), or decision-making, a gradual progression of assistance begins to be more obvious as family members or friends jump in and pick up the slack. Without much notice, family members, especially spouses, will eventually take on a household responsibility or do simple tasks for the person, thinking perhaps the person is getting "lazy" in their "old age."

Assistance can be subtle, such as helping search for lost items or becoming the keeper of the television remote. It is easy in the early stage to unconsciously deny something is wrong and begin making excuses for your loved one's changes to your children, other family members, friends and neighbors, thus allowing yourself time to make sense of the changes. We want to protect our loved one, but if friends and family members do not have a clear understanding of dementia, they may see their loved one as "diminished" due to the cognitive decline, and they will treat the person "as if they were no longer a human being and in nonhuman ways." (16)

Minimizing changes in your loved one can buy time to begin accepting the changes in your life that a dementia diagnosis will bring. This denial can be helpful for a little while; however, once you come to terms with yourself and realize your loved one requires extra daily support due to a neuro-cognitive disorder, the sooner you can learn strategies to keep the person independent longer, cognitive can slow down. With the continuous responsibilities of juggling home life and often balancing a work life, you may perhaps become less focused on your life and more on someone else's. If that happens, losing your own personhood or sense of self can result. Does taking on the role of a "caregiver" become your purpose in life, or is caregiving actually a responsibility that does not define you?

As memory loss and confusion progresses in your loved one, maintaining your "self" is vital. Research has shown that "loss of self" for spouses and adult children caring for a family member with dementia is common, especially for females, and this loss of identity is a result of "engulfment in the caregiver role." Lack of social contacts outside of the family is tied to a greater loss of self and is associated with depression and lower self-esteem. (17).

During times of caregiving, and even after caregiving ends, either through death or an alternative living setting for your loved one, family members and friends may feel lost and perceive they "do not know who they are anymore." The death of a spouse, sister, brother, parent, or friend, under any circumstance, may evoke a feeling to question if a life with meaning without that person is even possible. But with a healthy sense of self, even when the pain of grief seems unbearable, your personal identity does not have to change. The core of our being lives in our hearts.

A woman and her husband, who had dementia, participated in one of my dyadic groups for over two years. He was in his eighties and passed away from cancer. They had been married for over sixty years, raising two children and living a life filled with travel and adventures. A couple of weeks following his death, I received an email from her asking for my help. She told me she had never lived alone and needed to learn how to live without her husband.

Transition periods of an unwanted or unexpected change can be difficult, but in the book *How to Survive Change You Didn't Ask For*, MJ Ryan suggests that "fear is the true challenge of change." She encourages you to "remind yourself of your accomplishments." Much like tapping into your Superpowers that helped you get through difficult times in the past, discovering your hidden strengths can give you the resilience to navigate change a bit easier.

After meeting with the woman who asked for my help to learn to live alone without her husband, we discovered her fear was based on the reality that she did not just lose a beloved spouse; she lost her lifelong leisure partner. She and her husband enjoyed plays, concerts, trips to the museum, volunteer work and numerous other activities. Her efforts to keep them both engaged in a meaningful life were remarkable throughout the time I knew them. It turned out she did have a strong sense of self and began attending activities alone, inviting friends, spending more time with her children, traveling and eventually discovering new ways to live a meaningful life again.

Building a strong sense of self by setting healthy boundaries, asking for help, and increasing self-awareness to gain insight into how you think, value, and feel about yourself gives direction to your life. Being able to "quiet" the negative self-talk we often have when we feel pulled in many directions, our ability to adjust goals to live a life of purpose if our self-identity is being compromised.

Participating in activities, whether enjoying the outdoors, playing cards, reading, art or exercising, expressing ourselves through our hobbies helps make daily life meaningful and brings happiness. Remember the joy you feel when you engage in an activity that is interesting and fun? How long has it been since you have been caring for your loved one? Have you given yourself permission to enjoy life, if even for a few minutes? We have to give ourselves permission to "play" and enjoy recreation, even when going through difficult times. Recreation means to "re-create" a positive feeling, emotion, or experience. You may have your own health barriers that limit what you would like to be doing, but you have the capacity to adjust goals and live a life with purpose and meaning.

Someone living with memory loss, confusion, and poor motivation, however, is unable to shift a goal or identify new goals and maintain the direction in their life. Initiating an activity that used to be enjoyable, such as golf, cooking, or even grilling out, becomes problematic. When you make a commitment to support your family member or friend in the home, the responsibility of offering and engaging with your loved one with meaningful activities that can bring them joy falls to you. Not always you personally, but inviting other family members, neighbors, or friends to be an integral part of your loved one's life. The less interaction and stimulation a person has in general, the greater the risk for depression and faster cognitive decline occurs.

Practicing how to adapt tasks/activities for the person's changing abilities and needs by always focusing on what they can do, not what they cannot do, is a strengths-based approach to providing quality care. Connecting with your loved one and ensuring success is the real meaning of the activity and helps your loved one feel purpose and self-worth. Making the task easy at times is appropriate; however, don't be afraid to adapt a task or activity to be a bit challenging. Accomplishing difficult tasks encourages all of us to feel a greater sense of accomplishment.

From the earliest hint that something is "just not right," and prior to any official diagnosis of a neuro-cognitive disorder, such as dementia or Alzheimer's disease, the person's quality of life is affected, as is yours. Social, behavioral, cognitive and sometimes physical changes occur and influence the person and their family and friends' perception of a reduced sense of purpose. This perception can lead to depression, anxiety, shame, paranoia, and social withdrawal in the person experiencing the changes and those who love them. Thus, it is imperative families and friends support the person in maintaining purpose and meaning in each day and share joyful moments. Research indicates that the person living with dementia feel that staying connected with others improves their quality of life and contributes to living well.

Because of changes in the brain, internal motivation can lessen, and the person may appear disinterested in life. This may also be a result of the person realizing the slow loss of independence they are experiencing, such as driving restrictions or the inability to initiate, plan and execute activities and hobbies they used to enjoy. Family members and friends may conclude the person is unable to do the activity any longer or has completely lost interest, and the family just writes it off "as part of having dementia." This usually is not the case, however, especially during the early stages of dementia. Lifestyle adaptations and respectful support to stay engaged in life and maintain a sense of belonging and is an important considerations. Inaccurate assumptions and negative reactions to early dementia can result in low expectations of the person's actual abilities and have a greater impact on the long-term health outcomes for the person and the family.

Creating areas in your home that invite activities, such as keeping bird feeders full and hung by a window with chairs and binoculars handy, supports the "self" and allows someone to continue enjoying the backyard birds. Something as simple as making the piano easily accessible and the seat not filled with "stuff," the pianist can sit and play at will or perhaps with encouragement from you. Building raised garden beds so a gardener can feel the soil and remember the good times of raising a vegetable or flower garden, or bring out the old albums and "record player" stashed away and dance or sing together.

Music today, of course, is much more advanced and crisper than the old 33 albums, but there is something about that crackling sound I still enjoy. I spoke earlier of the woman with "no interest in stamp collecting" and seeing no value in sitting with her husband so he might enjoy a past interest. Creating engagement is not always about you, and creating shared joyful moments is as important. Understanding and feeling the value and power of connectedness, relationships, and purpose is really the desired outcome when engaging with anyone.

For someone to live with purpose, contributing to conversations and decisions is very important. Imagine how frustrating it would be to sit in a room with people speaking a language you do not understand. People with dementia must feel the same kind of frustration when people around them discuss current events because it is difficult for someone with confusion to follow conversations and process new information. Because past memories remain stored in our brains the longest, sharing stories of a better time, often repeating the same story, even during one conversation, gives purpose to the person experiencing memory loss. By validating that wonderful memory each time the story is told, we empower the person to continue to feel connected and relevant with purpose. Studies show a correlation between greater purpose in life and lower rates of depression.

Many people struggle to find purpose, and according to Larissa Rainey, an Organizational Psychology Researcher, some people actually experience "purpose anxiety," experiencing negative emotions in relation to the search for purpose. She suggests the solution isn't to search more "But appreciate what you have." She says our purpose lives inside us.

When people begin to experience cognitive and physical changes, a void in life's meaning can result in searching for purpose. People living with dementia can have periods of high anxiety, and families may insist the doctor "treat" that symptom with medication. But I wonder if people with dementia are having symptoms similar to those of "purpose anxiety," seeking their purpose for that day or even moment.

Communicating unmet needs through actions, such as roaming throughout the house with no predetermined destination, rummaging through drawers hoping to discover something to do or searching for something they hid for safekeeping and cannot recall where they placed the item. I was working with a family who shared with me that their mother, who was living with dementia, "escaped" from the house (the first time) and was found almost a mile away, walking on the side of a highway. When she was located, she was surprised to see her son and explained she was "going to the store to get milk to help him out." Implementing the L.O.V.E. Approach and taking time to listen and recognize her unmet need to feel helpful, rather than interpreting her "escape" as nefarious, can give you an opportunity to validate that need and engage in activities that will bring meaning.

Wanting to feel helpful and useful for someone having difficulty demonstrating logical thinking and organizing thoughts often results in repetitive actions and items going missing in the house. Moving or hiding objects (a man who continually searches for his misplaced wallet) is a coping mechanism to make sense of the confusing world a person now lives in or an attempt to try to gain some control over their situation. There is always a logical reason in the person's mind for hiding or moving objects, but it makes little sense to us until we learn to listen and observe. Thus, being mindful there is always intent. Finding missing cookies in the pantry with the dog food, although annoying, the intent was commendable because the person was likely just putting the cookies away. Avoid scolding the person for an action that seemed logical; just move the cookies back where they belong.

Creating meaningful activities can create purpose and improve the mood and sense of self for your loved one. It will also decrease "dementia symptoms" that can manifest because of boredom, anxiety, or just lack of stimulation. Keeping your family member involved in meal prep, self-care, or a familiar hobby is very important. Because of a decrease in initiating activities, setting the person up for success is key. Meaningful activities should be linked to hobbies or tasks that are related to previous work and can provide a person living with dementia with emotionally nurturing experiences and increase self-esteem and feelings of validation. The skill level may not be as high as before dementia, so it is important to adapt activities to their current abilities. The purpose of engaging in an activity with someone living with dementia is the why, not the what.

While reading Priya Parker's book, *The Art of Gathering: How We Meet and Why It Matters*, I developed a deeper understanding of "gathering for a purpose." She suggests that we rarely think of the deeper meaning and purpose when planning a gathering, focusing on practicality such as decorations, music, or food. While Ms Parker was addressing actual physical gatherings such as parties, holidays, and weddings and defining a gathering of three or more people, the message to "think less about the what, and more about the why" really resonated with me.

A gentleman recently told me his last family gathering was noisy and chaotic, and he observed his father with dementia become overwhelmed and upset along with other family members, concluding the gathering was a "disaster." The family didn't realize the gathering was not about the number of family members who could get together and enjoy a meal, but the gathering was for connecting with each other in meaningful ways. Finding a quiet spot for his dad, inviting family members to visit one-on-one, and giving his father breaks from the noise and commotion would have perhaps resulted in a better outcome.

In her book, Ms Parker defines a gathering as three people and suggests the importance of a "human experience" as why we gather. Having worked in addiction, I learned an Alcoholics Anonymous (AA) meeting can consist of just two alcoholics joining to support each other in sobriety.

So I began thinking more about a gathering of just two people, such as a person living with dementia and a family member or friend and the importance of the "human experience."

The next time you and your friend or family member are doing something together, whether preparing a salad, riding in a golf cart, taking a walk, or sitting and listening to music, remember it is not about meal preparations, golf, exercise or singing a song. Think less of what you are doing and more about the why and the human experience of that intimate gathering. This reinforces feelings of purpose.

Why does your loved one living with memory loss and confusion need to maintain purpose, and how can you support that need? Let's look at a task we have all done throughout our lives: getting dressed each morning. The overall goal of getting dressed is to be ready for the day; however, your purpose for the task may be for your loved one to get the clothes on quickly because there are many daily responsibilities to tackle or the person has a doctor's appointment and you are running behind.

On the other hand, the purpose of dressing for the person may be to accomplish this task with the least amount of assistance and feel independent and generally not in a hurry, and the amount of time it may take is not a factor. To that person, it is the process that matters. Objectives (the small steps to achieve the goal) are needed, such as choosing the clothes and putting on the clothes in the correct order. If you are in a hurry, you can choose the clothes more quickly and dress the person in record time. Oftentimes, there is resistance from the person to accept assistance, and the routine task of dressing each morning can result in an upsetting conflict. Usually, if you don't insist, the person will not resist when accomplishing any task and delay the task and try it later.

Having your agenda (get dressed quickly) rather than the person's agenda (feel independent) can result in an imbalance of power addressed earlier in the book. Supporting the person's need to continue to live with purpose and meaning very much depends on your willingness to let the person do tasks, such as dressing, on their own. Please don't jump to a conclusion at this point and tell me that your loved one would put on a dirty shirt, not button it properly, and perhaps even put on two pairs of pants. The person lives with confusion; thus, assistance is needed to accomplish the goal of dressing, but not doing it for the person but with the person. Learning to be flexible and taking a moment to adjust goals to adapt to a situation when that goal is no longer realistic may not be easy; however, it is a positive step toward achieving the desired outcome and an opportunity for your personal growth.

Minimizing the clothes to choose from will be helpful for the person in making a decision. Only have perhaps three or four of the person's favorite shirts, dresses, shoes etc, in the closest so it won't be overwhelming. Handing each article of clothing one at a time and using subtle verbal, visual or physical prompts if needed will support their independence. Putting on socks and shoes seems fairly simple; however, motor planning, visual perception, hand strength, grasp, and bilateral coordination, or the ability to use both sides of the body in a task or activity, is very complicated. Handing socks one at a time and then shoes one at a time will help minimize the complexity.

There are many nice-looking slip-on sneakers and even dress shoes that will eliminate the tying process of shoelaces and will still preserve the person's dignity. Adaptive clothes are also available and can make dressing easier. Using the L.O.V.E. Approach to listen and observe will help when adapting and breaking down the tasks as skill levels change and will make the engagement more meaningful and go smoother. Of course, your patience and encouragement will validate the person's efforts and promote well-being and dignity.

I hope the example above helps you to understand how the L.O.V.E. Approach works. The more you practice listening, observing, validating and engaging, these four concepts will be implemented in your interactions naturally. Once you begin to see the positive outcomes of this approach and understand why your loved one does what he/she does, even when it doesn't make sense to you, fewer conflicts will occur, and both of you can experience more joyful moments.

Communication is key, and being aware of what we say and how we say it can make a difference. So often, in passing, we may mention something that must get done, such as paying bills, or someone will visit soon or mentioning a 10:00 am doctor appointment that is two months away. Seems innocent enough; however, when a person is experiencing confusion, memory loss, and distortion of time, all of these examples can lead to unnecessary concern and result in expressed anxiety with frequent questions to reassure the person that he/she will not miss the event.

Staying in the present is key to minimizing stress in your loved one's life. The person will worry the doctor's appointment will be missed, or a bill is not paid. Asking repeatedly, "When is our son coming?" "What time is my doctor's appointment?" "Did you file the taxes?" will create anxiety for both of you. So, how do you create a more relaxed environment?

In the previous chapter, I suggested a need for a more balanced and "integrated holistic, humanistic, whole-body, family-centered and ecopsychosocial approach to supporting people living with dementia. Treating family members by addressing depression, anxiety, treat families along with the family member with dementia." I believe creating a family-friends-centered approach for the treatment of dementia is possible and can be effective in maintaining relationships, promoting independence and engaging in meaningful activities.

Often, activities such as music, massage, poetry, art, or dance are considered "non-pharmacological," but that term does not fully explain the benefits of these activities other than they do not involve a drug, describing what they are not rather than what they are. An ecopsychosocial approach for treating cognitive decline has evolved and encompasses community awareness, educational efforts for families, and social support for individuals who can improve functioning.

"The goal of this new label is to be better able to compare interventions and their outcomes and to be able to see the connections between data sets presently not seen as fitting together, thereby encouraging a greater focus on developing new ecopsychosocial interventions and approaches that can improve the lives of those with dementia, their care partners, and the broader society."(18)

Recognizing that not just the psycho-social needs are an important part of this concept, the environment or "eco" is also a needed consideration to promote inclusion and help reduce the stigma of dementia. The term ecopsychosocial interventions "focuses on learning communication techniques, teaching strategies for connectedness and engagement, and using a whole body approach by addressing the environment and the physical, cognitive, social, expressive and spiritual needs of the person and the family". Interventions can include music, exercise, visual arts, reminiscent therapy, and validation therapy, tapping into hobbies and meaningful activities, and many libraries, art classes, and community organizations are offering programs specific to persons living with cognitive in the hope of creating a more inclusive community.

*"We don't stop playing because we grow old; we grow old because we stop playing."*
– George Bernard Shaw

Many families find that developing a meaningful daily routine early into the diagnosis will make the progression of memory loss much easier. Begin the morning at breakfast ( yes, eat together) and perhaps share a daily scripture to engage in a conversation. Take a morning walk together and plan time during the day to enjoy music, dance, and sing.

The Global Action Plan on Dementia recognizes physical, cognitive and social activities can "maintain or improve functioning, interpersonal relationships and well-being" in people living with dementia.

As I mentioned earlier, I am not anti-drug, and medications for managing pain are crucial. Pain is a significant trigger of behavioral disturbances in dementia patients but is often overlooked or ignored. A study showed more than half of the patients with dementia in hospitals experience daily pain. For people living with dementia, pain can often be attributed to an increase in dementia symptoms such as crying, apathy, depression, or suddenly lacking the motivation to participate to engage in activities. Because some people with dementia are unable to express with words they have pain, assessing pain can be difficult. You may recall from an earlier chapter that all behaviors are a means to communicate an unmet need and can result in changes in your loved one's mood. Pain in people with dementia is increasingly recognized as both under-assessed and under-treated.

Learning how to validate your family member's feelings, avoiding correcting your loved one on inaccurate facts, and allowing the person to have purpose and meaning in their life by reminiscing events can make for a much more pleasant and less stressful day. These approaches are not only helpful to the person living with memory loss but also a natural way for the family members or friends providing care to take care of their own well-being and improve their quality of life.

Unlike medications that have side effects and " work in some "people," there are no downsides or side effects to trying ecopsychosocial interactions with a person living with dementia. Activities can be adapted to meet the person where they are and to their ability levels. And unlike the medications that may help with some symptoms, your family member's needs are not being addressed. With meaningful and fun activities, both you and your family members can enjoy the benefits of engagement.

Our perceptions of people with dementia matter. I recently saw a post on my neighborhood app by someone referring to his neighbor as a "dementia patient." In the context of a physician, the person is a "patient," but to everyone else, the person is a person. Family members will refer to their loved one as a "patient," reinforcing their belief the person is sick rather than living with a disability.

The person living with dementia remains your friend or family member even if the person transitions into assisted living or another community and is only a patient to the doctor or nurses. That imbalance of power is more prevalent when a friend or family sees the family as a "patient" rather than humanizing the person as a spouse or parent and creates the mindset of "caregiving" and doing for the person rather than with the person. The person is a person, not a patient, when you are a friend or family member.

Teachable moments offer awareness and help in breaking stigma, and like the mother in the grocery store who passed judgment on me and the little boy with autism, this seemed like an opportunity for a teachable moment about the perceptions of people with dementia, so I politely commented. His response was an emphatic, "I don't care."

Close minded people don't want their beliefs challenged and are unwilling to consider other viewpoints regardless of evidence the information is accurate. When it comes to changing the beliefs and a preconceived bias regarding an issue, open minded people tend to believe their belief may be wrong and will ask questions rather than making statements to support their belief. This is why it is so important for all of us to educate, advocate and encourage others to see people living with dementia as people with feelings, not as an "epidemic".

## Activity 1

Research shows how we played as a child sets us up for how we behave as an adult in all domains. List childhood play activities (riding a bike, sports, swimming, collecting things, making things, learning things).

## Activity 2

List your current hobbies, interests, and activities and compare them to your childhood list. Any similarities?

## Activity 3

Write down messages you received as a child from parents, teachers, or others about play and explore if those messages hold true to your value of play or recreation today.

Example: Negative play messages:
- Sundays are for rest, not play.
- You have to be quiet when you play.
- There is no time for play.

Positive play messages
- Have fun!
- You are so creative!
- Stay safe

## Activity 4

It is never too late to develop your playful, humorous side, even when times are tough. Feeling self-conscious and fearing embarrassment or negative messages from your childhood can limit your ability to be more playful. Name three things you are willing to try the next week (even if this may feel uncomfortable) to practice a more relaxed and playful side.

# Activity 5

Write about your purpose in life.

# Chapter 10
## Friends, Family and Faith

*"To the world you may be one person; but to one person you may be the world."*
-Dr. Seuss

## Friends

Some friends in our lives are friends by circumstance, such as when a couple shares friends during a relationship. However, if circumstances change, such as a breakup or death of one of the couples, some circumstantial friendships may end. However, a "true friend" comes into our lives, and despite all the shortcomings and changes we experience, they never leave. My childhood friend, for example, was a circumstantial friend because I lived next door to her growing up, but despite moving apart and leading separate lives, we are friends by choice today and have enjoyed our friendship for over sixty years.

Friends matter and are important throughout our lives. Friendships in early childhood give a sense of belonging and social identity, and studies find early childhood friends contribute to a child's quality of life. As adults, friendships continue to be important, adding fun to our lives and providing emotional support, especially during difficult times. When a friend learns of a friend's dementia diagnosis, a reaction of shock may be the first response, usually because of the lack of understanding of the diagnosis and concern about how it will affect the friendship. Wondering what to say or do can cause apprehension to stay connected. Just remember your friendship was built on common interests; perhaps you are both fathers, grandfathers, athletes, mothers, singers, or hikers.

When a friend doesn't understand dementia or the changes a friend is experiencing, it can be intimidating. Shifting the way you will experience the relationship and wondering if this can be a priority for you may cause feelings of ambiguity in maintaining the friendship. Even being fearful of the changes in the person is very common and normal. Utilizing the L.O.V.E. Approach by listening, observing, validating, and engaging in common interests with your friend allows you to withstand the changes and maintain a reciprocal friendship. The family can be helpful in sharing effective engagement techniques and help you to interact with your friends more easily. Regular phone calls are a great way to start reaching out and maintain the relationship.

I believe most friends want to continue the friendship, even after a diagnosis, but may not know how. I think of these individuals as "true friends." Friends for life who are committed to maintaining the social connection and accepting each other without judgment and with mutual respect. Often, a close friend may be the first to notice subtle changes as the person begins to experience cognitive decline, such as forgetting recent events, talking off-topic or forgetting lunch dates.

One of the reasons friends become friends is because of shared interests. Think of your friends and the activities you enjoy together. You may have a walking buddy and another friend you count on for lunch dates or afternoons at the theatre, or perhaps one best friend who shares all these activities. "Purposeful connections, and engaging in meaningful activities with other people, are important to a person with dementia and their families/care providers." (19)

Friends greatly influence opportunities for leisure engagement, as leisure activities often require planning and social resources. "One of the main factors affecting social engagement opportunities for individuals with dementia is having friends who stop calling or visiting when they learn about their dementia diagnosis." (20)

"True friends" are also very important for the person providing the care of a loved one with dementia to stay connected. So many of the families feel their friends do not stay in touch but are reluctant to reach out for fear they are a bother. And much like the ambiguity felt with the friends of the person with dementia, these friends may need a little direction on how to help.

In one of the summer camps I managed for children with autism, I had an intern who was a bit fearful of one older camper. He didn't speak and would suddenly stand up and run around the gymnasium with long strides, leaping much like a graceful deer in the forest, oblivious to everything else. She was startled by this sudden burst of energy, and it made her reluctant to engage with him.

I explained to my young intern that he was just meeting his need for physical activity and self-expression, and running made him very happy. The next couple of days, I recollect her observing him closely while in the gym and can recall so vividly the first time she joined his world. He suddenly jumped up to begin his usual laps in the gym, and I saw her stand up from the bleachers and run to catch up with him.

Once she was leaping beside him, she reached for his hand. It was almost magical. He turned and looked at her, grasping her hand firmly and encouraging her to join him, almost like synchronized dancers. Hand in hand and leaping joyfully together, she rounded the curve with her new friend, giving me a big smile, a thumbs up and a triumph shout, "I get him now!" This is a great example of the L.O.V.E. Approach and the importance of embracing the personhood of your friend with dementia and focusing on the psychosocial needs, especially the need for human connections with your friend.

Joining your friend living in a world of confusion will make a significant difference, not just to the person, but to you. A friend who stays connected in a relationship with a friend with dementia will grow personally in unexpected ways. However, understanding the unmet needs and the reactions your friend may have if a need is not being met is key to maintaining a meaningful relationship.

The intern who "got him" observed the young camper's routine to better understand his needs, validated those needs by running with him, and took a risk to explore if he had any other needs. By offering her hand as they ran, he also had a need to engage with her through physical touch. The willingness of this young intern to take in new information and shift her paradigm from the belief this camper was unpredictable and began believing he was a child communicating his needs by joyfully running evolved into a wonderful relationship. Her intentional effort to observe and meet his needs allowed him to engage more easily, sharing his joy with others throughout the summer.

Remember my friend who modified the golfing experience with her friend by transitioning from putting green to simply riding around the course in a golf cart when holding a club became too difficult? She chose to be a "true friend," knowing their friendship was too important, recognizing it wasn't about playing golf but the true purpose of the "gathering."

If your friend has a dementia diagnosis, and if you haven't already connected, I encourage you to reach out today, even with just a quick phone call. Your friend needs the reassurance of human connections and to continue contributing to your friendship. If it has been a long friendship, storytelling and reminiscing about the early years will come naturally. Be mindful of not correcting your friend when stories are inaccurate, and just listen, smile and enjoy your time together, even when stories are repeated. To encourage your friend to tell a story, prompt with "I recall" or "I was thinking about" and avoid asking, if they "remember" an event or a person. This approach can create a positive and meaningful engagement, unlike the embarrassment and shame the proud Marine felt after being corrected by his wife on his discharge date from the military.

Maintaining your friend's dignity and autonomy is an amazing way to honor the person's living legacy (purpose and contributions) and help to build their life legacy (values, beliefs, hopes and dreams) left for their loved ones. Creating a memory box with your friend and including pictures from the past and items to hold that may help your friend retrieve memories can be helpful as dementia progresses. For example, if fishing was an activity you enjoyed in the past, using a small tackle box as the memory box would be ideal. If you and your friend enjoy sewing, use a sewing box and include pictures, fabric squares to feel, ribbons or spools of thread. Rummaging through the boxes when you are together and adding other items that evoke memories can be very engaging. Keeping the box and sharing it when you are together helps your friend to associate these items with your friendship and can help to reduce any subtle stress for both of you.

I hope you choose to be "true friends" for life because your friend misses the friendship, and I can guess you miss having that person in your life as well. If you don't include your friend in your life, you may regret it later on. If you search online for "treatment for dementia," you will likely see the emphasis is the pharmacological approach. I believe, however, that friends are one of the best "treatments" to improve the quality of life and overall well-being of someone living with dementia. You may be a little apprehensive about reaching out, but the more you understand your friend and insights into your growth, going out for coffee or just sitting on the porch to visit may feel like old times. It certainly would for your friend.

## Family

I have found relationships with friends are less stressful than family relationships; I think it's because friends are a bit more forgiving of blunders or gaffes. It is not surprising that family members may have high levels of stress as they spend the most time with the person, and the person becomes their center of attention. Family members who care for someone with dementia are more susceptible to developing adverse health outcomes.

In chapter three, when introducing the four concepts of the L.O.V.E. Approach, I used the quote by Lao Tzu that proposes if you give a man a fish, you feed him for a day as it makes sense to teach the skill so he would never be hungry again. The L.OV.E. Approach teaches you to listen, observe, validate and engage, giving you the tools to problem-solve situations as they arise. But let's consider the man you want to teach to fish is starving. Is this a good time to teach the skill, or should you just give him a fish to ease his hunger pain? I say, just give the man a fish!

When a family member providing constant care is having a difficult time, it is not the time for advice, criticism, or judgment. Like the starving man, give the family member the metaphorical fish to ease their emotional pain. Listen closely without responding initially. Silence and your presence can be powerful. You may hear a recurring theme, such as lack of sleep or a feeling of hopelessness because some issue has never been properly addressed. Most people just want someone to just be with them for a while. Being quiet and listening without judgment and with empathy, "imagine" how the person may feel in their current situation.

Observe and identify if an unmet need may be causing the person's distress. Is the loved one's dementia progressing, or does the house need a good cleaning? Also, observe your body language. Did you immediately stop what you were doing or roll your eyes and continue playing on your phone, missing an opportunity to show sincere concern? Look around and see if "an elephant is in the room." Is the loved one's hygiene overlooked, and perhaps a shower or clean clothing is needed?

Validate the person's feelings. Emotional neglect is hurtful and can feel like manipulation when a person's feelings are dismissed, minimized or not even acknowledged. You may think the feelings are silly or the person is just sensitive; for that person, their reality is what is important. You don't have to agree with the feelings, but refraining from solving the "problem" validates the person, as they may not see the situation as a problem to be solved but rather as a feeling that needs to be affirmed.

Engage with the person by holding their hand or offering a gentle touch on the arm. Continue to engage after the person has become calm and perhaps invite the person to have a fresh cup of coffee or go for a short walk if possible. Feeling connected with the people we love is essential for healthy relationships.

Family members, neighbors, and friends (and even strangers in a grocery store) may try to give advice, trying to influence the type of care and decisions you are making for your loved one. Being more empathetic and showing compassion when the person caring for a loved one may be feeling the intense losses that come with a dementia diagnosis. Offering unhelpful opinions is not very productive.

The critics and the judges need to recognize when a family member is struggling, exhausted, overwhelmed, and perhaps losing self-confidence, the person needs help, not harm. The person may be overwhelmed with grief from the losses the person feels, especially the loss of the companionship and support of their loved one who used to help problem-solve, and have meaningful conversations. But because of the cognitive decline, the person is unable to show empathy and ease your pain. It is difficult and sometimes uncomfortable to respond to a person's grief, and no one can fix it or even understand it because grief is very personal, very real, and unique to that person.

Choosing a career in healthcare and as a young clinician out of college, I discovered grief was all around me, and I wasn't fully prepared for the losses of so many of my clients. Not only did I not know how to support my client's grief, I lacked the ability to process that grief for myself and create healthy professional boundaries. Professors may spend time preparing young healthcare professionals on the importance of understanding grief today, and if they don't, they should, but when I was in school, it was not addressed.

Beginning my career working in a "nursing home," it wasn't unusual for a resident to attend a morning class and by afternoon had passed away. I also did not consider the suicides and overdoes that would take the lives of kids I rock climbed or rode horses with the week before, during my work in alcohol and drug rehabilitation with adolescents. Even when working in the community, supporting parents as they processed the initial grief felt when they had a child with a congenital disability was totally unexpected.

I now have a much better understanding of the feelings of the loss felt in grief. With training, I facilitate drum circles for parents with the loss of a child, offer expressive arts sessions for veterans with PDST and grieving the loss of a limb, and now, support families living with the grief and realities of dementia. Personally, the grief I experienced in anticipation of my mother's death due to a chronic illness was overwhelming. During the years my mother was so ill, especially the three years prior to her death, every time the phone rang, my emotions immediately jumped to the thought this was the call to inform me my life would change. I was not prepared for the intense pain and profound feelings of sadness for her, me, and my family that came in waves and unexpected moments while my mom was still living.

Several years after my mother's death, I learned this type of grief had a name, and I was experiencing "anticipatory grief," defined as "the time between receiving a terminal diagnosis and death, filled with sorrow, anxiety, uncertainty and fear." (21) My years of grieving with the anticipation my mom would die however, did not lessen the blow when her actual death occurred. It was still an enormous shock, and I wasn't prepared for that kind of grief either. Teaching effective coping techniques to clients experiencing grief has been a necessary skill in my work, and I have learned to understand how grief affects a particular situation, a person, families, and me.

Because of losses such as retirement dreams, future plans, and the loss of companionship a dementia diagnosis brings, on top of the inability of the person with dementia to be able to understand these changes and discuss these issues with a loved one, "dementia grief" is completely different and any other grief. Dementia grief is "a distinctive type of grief, whereby the dependent or loved one is still physically 'present' but emotionally disconnected from the caregiver." (21)

"What distinguishes dementia grief from the anticipatory grief elicited by most other terminal medical conditions is the reduced opportunity to experience relationship resolution between the informal carers and the person with dementia as well as share feelings about the compounded serial losses and impending death." (22)

It is difficult to detach from grief, but perhaps finding a safe place for your grief to rest at times can bring some solitude. Grief is internal, and mourning is the outward sign of grief. I am currently coaching a woman whose husband has dementia, and after two years of learning of his diagnosis, she cried for the first time this week.

## Faith

Spiritual connectedness is key to our overall well-being. This is especially true for persons living with memory loss and their families. Creating and sharing moments that promote spiritual growth can improve overall happiness and quality of life for all. Not only is this nurturing the spirit of personhood, but it also brings opportunities to maintain relationships with friends and family.

Spirituality is very personal and can have different meanings, but basically, it is a search to find purpose, meaning, and connectedness in your life. Studies show when those needs are not met, a person with dementia is at greater risk for depression, anxiety, an increase in physical pain, a lower sense of well-being and a decline in a life of quality. The L.O.V.E. Approach can help recognize these unmet needs. Listening and observing to understand purposeful behaviors by your loved one that make no sense to us, such as rummaging through drawers and closets. Perhaps consider this as a search for a Bible or another item that brings comfort and a sense of peace.

Despite a person's confusion and difficulty retrieving memories, the person retains the ability to feel and respond to emotions. The person with dementia may have difficulty expressing spiritual needs, but finding ways to help the person sense and feel their spiritual connection is important. To my knowledge, there is no evidence to suggest spiritual needs are lessened for people living with Alzheimer's disease or any other type of dementia. Unfortunately, spiritual needs are often overlooked and even dismissed, which can cause spiritual distress or the inability to find sources of love, hope, and connections for what is happening in their life.

Understanding the person has difficulty with thinking and reasoning, it is up to us to create opportunities for individuals to own and express their spiritual needs. Dementia affects the mind and body, and many see the person as an "empty shell," but I don't think the soul is compromised. I believe many of the concerning actions of the person are attempts to meet the unmet need to seek peace and calm, and we need to assist in their search. "When individuals face the uncertainties of advanced, terminal illness, as they do in the case of dementia, they may turn to religion or spirituality to cope." (23)

Many people find a connectedness to spirituality in nature. Walking outdoors and taking in the smells, sights and sounds or watching sunrises and sunsets and grasping the beauty of nature can be healing. Author Mary H. Frakes, a new friend of mine, wrote a beautiful book, *MindWalks*, as a way to encourage others to walk mindfully to relieve stress, inspire motivation, and nurture the soul by capturing the world around you. Originally published in 1999, Frakes was a visionary. She introduced "mindfulness," or a type of walking meditation, before "mindfulness" was even popular. Walking mindfully and staying in the present can lift your spirit and reach your inner self. It takes practice to stay in the moment and embrace your surroundings, and each walk will be a different experience, but it is well worth it when you find yourself feeling tranquil and centered.

Other nontraditional spiritual practices include relaxation, visualization, drumming, yoga, and guided imagery. Running, gardening, or participating in any activity with earth-grounding potential can also feed your spirit. Although spirituality is not always considered in healthcare, it is thought to play a role in positive health outcomes and healing. Compassionate care and a holistic approach, using evidence-based physical, social, cognitive, expressive (emotional) and spiritual activities, can improve your health, life satisfaction, and overall happiness and well-being.

But what about faith? Faith is different in people, and I think faith is believing in something that may not be easily believed or understood. And what about hope? Is hope what gives us the confidence to look toward our future, or does hope support the belief in our faith? Remember the small blue locomotive that believed she could pull a large train over a mountain even though the odds were against her? Was it her hope she could accomplish the feat or her faith that she believed she could cross the mountain? I have heard that faith will move mountains, or in this case, perhaps her belief in herself helped her overcome the hurdle of that mountain.

I also believe faith is the ability to believe in ourselves. Faith in ourselves means we have self-confidence, self-trust, self-respect and autonomy. We believe we can overcome doubt and accomplish things we have never done before, which leads us back to hoping things will be ok. The self-efficacy skills we addressed in chapter seven are key to learning new skills. If we stop believing in ourselves, we are unable to flourish, and we are at risk of losing the zest in life and stopping the things that bring us joy.

Remember the man who painted his self-portrait holding a balloon and floating in the air? When he explained he felt as if he was floating, perhaps he was letting us know he did not feel grounded in his faith. When we lose trust in ourselves and live with self-doubt, the results can lead to serious health consequences and a feeling of a lost identity. While struggling years ago when a pivotal moment changed the direction of my life, I never lost faith or hope. Having faith and hope can give you the ability to live positively, even during difficult times.

## Activity 1

You will need colored pencils and a piece of paper for this activity.

In spiritual rituals, hands are associated with prayer and blessings. We use our hands to greet people, to say hello and goodbye, and to clap to show appreciation. Hands can also represent strength and generosity by "lending a hand." This expressive art activity can help you find new depths to thinking and feeling that can apply these insights to all areas of life.

Individually or as a family, trace both your left and right-hand side by side on one piece of paper. Using words or symbols (anything you want) and in the traced left hand, identify things you have lost during this time of your life, such as dreams or companionship. In your right hand, identify represents what you can give and receive and things you want to hold on to, such as faith, friends, and good health.

## Activity 2

You will need a piece of paper, scissors and a pencil or pen.

Value clarification is a process to identify core values that influence our actions, emotions, decisions, and thoughts.

Cut the piece of paper into ten or twelve strips and write one value on each strip of paper (something important to you that influences the way you see yourself and the world). Place the strips in a column according to their priority to you. For example, if faith is the core belief, it will be at the top. Values can change according to circumstances. You can make two copies of your strips and make one column of your priorities to think back before the dementia diagnosis. Have they changed?

# Activity 3

Are you ready to try new strategies to support your loved one? Name three changes you are committed to implement

# Activity 4

Please complete the post-evaluation below and then compare it to the pre-evaluation you completed in Chapter One. Are you pleased with the results?

<u>Post-evaluation of knowledge, awareness, attitudes and values</u>

Please circle the response that best describes you.

| | | | | |
|---|---|---|---|---|
| 1. Understanding dementia is | poor | fair | good | great |
| 2. Ability to care for my loved one | poor | fair | good | great |
| 3. Skills needed to provide care | poor | fair | good | great |
| 4. Confidence to provide care | poor | fair | good | great |
| 5. The belief I need to learn new skills | poor | fair | good | great |
| 6. Importance of my needs | poor | fair | good | great |
| 7. My motivation to change | poor | fair | good | great |
| 8. I value myself, and my needs | poor | fair | good | great |
| 9. Knowledge of dementia symptoms | poor | fair | good | great |
| 10. Believe that recreation is important | poor | fair | good | great |
| 11. Confidence this book will help me | poor | fair | good | great |
| 12. My social support is | poor | fair | good | great |

# Conclusion

*"There is no greater agony than bearing an untold story inside of you."*
-Maya Angelou

Recalling and sharing memories from earlier times keeps us feeling alive and engaged in life. Stories are important because these memories build connections, invite conversations, elicit powerful emotions, and create feelings of happiness, especially for someone living with dementia. A person with memory loss will repeat their stories with the same enthusiasm as if it was being told for the first time, not remembering the story was told just moments before.

These stories will eventually fade, and when someone is stifled from sharing a meaningful memory, the person feels devalued, and the stories may suddenly stop. Listening and validating cherished memories helps the person to maintain their personhood and integrity. These meaningful memories need to be shared. Hearing repeated stories is taxing, but practicing listening with smiles, touch, and a playful heart, these stories build trust and deepen your relationship.

This book is more than introducing a holistic approach to treating dementia; but also about recognizing the importance of addressing your needs. The book offers an opportunity for you to develop a deeper understanding of how a dementia diagnosis affects you and thus will help you understand how dementia is affecting your loved one. Developing self-awareness and self-efficacy skills and practicing self-determination will help you believe in yourself. Recognizing your strengths, talents, and gifts and gaining an awareness of what motivates you will help to understand the essence of who you are. Your confidence and conviction to make the best decisions and provide optimal care for your loved one becomes apparent.

Having self-awareness is important in understanding who you are, your needs and what inspires and motivates you. Defining those "and then" or pivotal moments in your life, expected or unexpected, and especially those that are unwanted, will prompt you to do some soul-searching and better know yourself and how dementia is affecting you. Making a conscious effort to reflect on your responses to that pivotal moment can make you stronger than you realize. The L.O.V.E. Approach can make a difference as you become a more confident decision-maker.

Some decisions, of course, will be harder than others, and there may come a time when your family member requires more support than you can safely provide at home. Deciding to transition your loved one into a residential care community that can provide that support will likely be the hardest decision in your life, but it is the right thing to do for you and your family. Finding the setting that best meets the needs of your family member is key and may take time. To ensure the people who will now provide the care and compassion know that dementia is only part of your loved one's life, write the person's life story and post it in the room, encouraging connections and a person-centered care approach. This decision can feel like a betrayal, and you may be overwhelmed with guilt, feeling you have made a mistake and "gave up on the person you love," but it is a selfless act and adjusting does take time. I have yet to work with a family who did not eventually realize this was the best decision for their family.

Understanding your beliefs, feelings, and values allows you to live your best life, even in times of stress. Valuing our whole selves helps to remind us we are not perfect, but we are human beings doing the best we can with the courage to take risks, connect with others, and ask for help. If a value is not aligned with your lifestyle, a conflict will occur, causing stress and having a significant impact on your happiness and possibly your health. For example, if you value your health but are neglecting it by not exercising, eating or sleeping well, or keeping routine doctor appointments, an internal conflict will occur, and distress will follow.

By being true to yourself and confident in your identity, you can make a difference in the lives of others. During interactions in our daily lives, three things can happen: One, you will leave the interaction or conversation with a neutral outcome, and nothing significantly occurs with the other person. Secondly, you leave the interaction, and the person feels worse, or lastly, you leave the interaction, and the person feels better. This third outcome is the heart of the L.O.V.E. Approach. Although specifically developed for families caring for a loved one with dementia, listening, observing, validating and engaging with others will promote meaningful interactions in any situation. Stretching yourself and stepping out of your comfort zone into unfamiliar territories is scary, but change becomes easier each time you take a little risk and try something new. Change is both frightening and exciting. Are you ready? I believe you are.

While we wait on a cure or the next "groundbreaking approved drug," we lose time in keeping our family members as independent as possible and connecting with others. Medications may claim to extend the person's life. However, the person may not be living a life of quality. Medications cannot smile at your loved one or hold their hand for comfort and reassurance. Medications cannot sing or dance. Medications cannot listen to stories as the person tries to hold on to their personhood. And most importantly, medications cannot give a person meaning or purpose. I believe the best holistic treatment approach for dementia is people.

When we care for people holistically, we ensure we are not reducing our treatment approach to a single aspect of dementia. We step forward into action, which demonstrates an understanding and an acceptance of the multiple dimensions a person embodies. Therefore, a holism philosophy sees the bigger picture and appreciates the many dimensions of who a person is on the inside. Advocating for an integrated healthcare approach and providing support to individuals and families who live in a world of dementia today is my mission. I hope you will join me.

The song "Leaving on a Midnight Train to Georgia" sung by Gladys Knight and the Pips in the 1970's, to me is a beautiful allegory of a dementia journey. The song is about a man whose life in Los Angeles was too much for him, so he leaves his current life to find "the world he left behind not so long ago." He purchases a one-way ticket and leaves in the darkness for a train ride to "find a simpler time and place in his life." A commitment from someone who loves him and proclaims she will be by his side and would "rather live in his world than without him in mine" says it all. I have always loved this song because it comes from the perspective of someone who understands the pain someone is living and promises to be with them throughout the journey.

So, what does the future hold for your family and millions of others? I do not know, nor does anyone else, but I am hopeful things will change for the better. We are not promised a tomorrow, but if we practice living in the moment, becoming fully aware and attentive to that precious moment, life may seem a bit less overwhelming. Encouraging your family members to tell their stories, even in little inaccurate chunks, gives them the ability to communicate when daily conversation no longer makes sense. You also have stories to tell, and sharing yours is just as important. Times, places and characters in our loved ones' stories may be forgotten, and all stories will eventually end. You are now the keeper of those memories. Hold them close.

*"If there ever comes a day when we can't be together, keep me in your heart, and I'll stay there forever."* Winnie the Pooh

## References

1  Jopp DS, Schmitt M. Dealing with negative life events: differential effects of personal resources, coping strategies, and control beliefs.

2  Yang Y. Social inequalities in happiness in the United States, 1972 to 2004: an age-period-cohort analysis. Am Sociol Rev. 2008;73(2):204-226.

3  Watson R, Sanson-Fisher R, Bryant J, Mansfield E. Dementia is the second most feared condition among Australian health service consumers: results of a cross-sectional survey. BMC Public Health. 2023 May 12;23

4  Testing the efficacy of imagined contact and perspective-taking Jennifer Jiwon Na1, Alison L. Chasteen2 1Department of Psychology, University of British Columbia 2Department of Psychology, University of Toronto

5  National Institute on Aging. The study, led by Patricia Boyle at the Rush Alzheimer's Disease Research Center in Chicago, was published April 16 in Annals of Internal Medicine.

6  Zahed, S., Emami, M., Bazargan-Hejazi, S. et al. What motivates informal caregivers of people with dementia (PWD): a qualitative study. BMC Palliat Care 18, 105 (2019)

7  Engelman K, Altus DE, Mathews RM. Increasing engagement in daily activities by older adults with dementia. J Appl Behav Anal. 1999;32(1):107–110.

8  Pressman SD, Matthews KA, Cohen S, Martire LM, Scheier M, Baum A, Schulz R. Association of enjoyable leisure activities with psychological and physical well-being. Psychosom Med. 2009 Sep;71(7):725-32.

9  Cohen-Mansfield J, Dakheel-Ali M, Marx MS. Engagement in persons with dementia: the concept and its measurement. Am J Geriatr Psychiatry. 2009 Apr;17(4):299-307

10  Flannery RB Jr. Treating learned helplessness in the elderly dementia patient: preliminary inquiry. Am J Alzheimers Dis Other Demen. 2002 Nov-Dec;17

11  Miranda-Castillo, C., Woods, B. & Orrell, M. The needs of people with dementia living at home from user, caregiver and professional perspectives: a cross-sectional survey. BMC Health Survey

12  Montgomery and Kosloski 2009 Montgomery R. J. V, Kosloski K. (2009). Caregiving as a process of changing identity: Implications for caregiver support. Generations, 33(1), 47-52

13  Sabat SR. Capacity for decision making in Alzheimer's disease: selfhood, positioning and semiotic people. Aust N Z J Psychiatry. 2005;39:1030–1035.

14  Lee, S., Colditz, G. A., Berkman, L. F., & Kawachi, I. (2003). Caregiving and risk of coronary heart disease in U.S. women: A prospective study. American Journal of Preventive Medicine, 24(2), 113–119.

15  Yu DSF, Cheng S-T, Wang J. Unravelling positive aspects of caregiving in dementia: An integrative review of research literature. Int J Nurs Stud. 2018;79:1–26.

16  Fazio, S.(2008).The enduring self in people with Alzheimer's: Getting to the heart of individualized care.Baltimore, MD: Health Professions PressKitwood, T.,

&Bredin, K.(1992).Towards a theory of dementia care: Personhood and well-being.Ageing and Society,12,269–287.

17. Skaff MM, Pearlin LI. Caregiving: role engulfment and the loss of self. Gerontologist. 1992 Oct;32(5):656-64.

18. Ecopsychosocial Interventions in Cognitive Decline and Dementia: A New Terminology and a New Paradigm . / Zeisel, John; Reisberg, Barry; Whitehouse, Peter et al.In: American Journal of Alzheimer's Disease and Other Dementias, Vol. 31, No. 6, 01.09.2016, p. 502-507

19. Bruneau B. Barriers to the management of pain in dementia care. Nurs Times. 2014 Jul 9-15;110(28):12, 14-6.

20. Phinney A., Kelson E., Baumbusch J., OConnor D., Purves B. (2016). Walking in the neighbourhood: Performing social citizenship in dementia. Dementia, 15(3), 381–394

21. Rando TA. Rando T. A comprehensive analysis of anticipatory grief: Perspectives, processes, promises, and problems, Loss and anticipatory grief, 1986 New York Lexington Books(pg. 1-36)

22. Dehpour, T. , & Koffman, J. (2023). Assessment of anticipatory grief in informal caregivers of dependents with dementia: A systematic review. Aging & Mental Health, 27(1), 110–123

23. Blandin, K. , & Pepin, R. (2017). Dementia grief: A theoretical model of a unique grief experience. Dementia, 16(1), 67–78

24. Katsuno T. Personal spirituality of persons with early-stage dementia: is it related to perceived quality of life? Dementia. 2003;2(3):315-335

## About the Author

Vicky Pitner is a Certified Therapeutic Recreation Specialist, Certified Dementia Practitioner, consultant, national speaker, and an expert in dementia support. She weaves personal stories, metaphors, compelling research and anecdotes from her work experiences that lead to the L.O.V.E. Approach. She has been supporting children with neurodevelopmental disorders and adults with neurocognitive disorders for over forty years in both clinical and community settings. She shares her passions with anyone who will listen.

Made in the USA
Monee, IL
04 May 2026

49483519R00072